# 1001 little

# BEAUTY

# MIRACLES

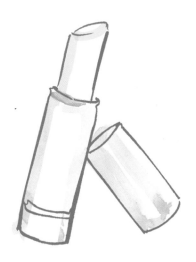

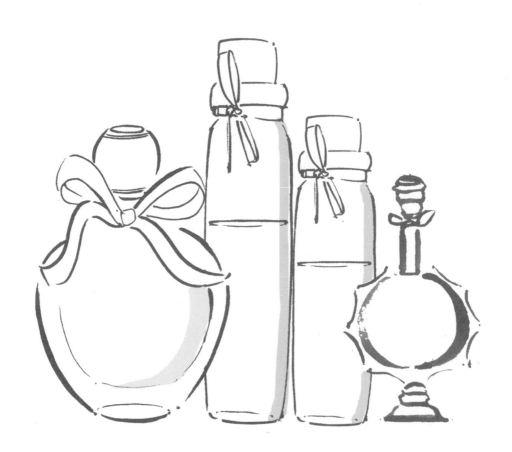

# 1001 little
# BEAUTY
# MIRACLES

## Secrets and solutions from head to toe

Esme Floyd

**CARLTON**
**BOOKS**

THIS IS A CARLTON BOOK

Text and design copyright © 2006
Carlton Books Limited

This edition published in 2011 by
Carlton Books Limited
20 Mortimer Street
London W1T 3JW

10 9 8 7 6 5 4 3 2 1

ISBN: 978 184732 952 3

Printed and bound in China

Senior Executive Editor: Lisa Dyer
Art Director: Lucy Coley
Design: Liz Wiffen
Copy Editor: Libby Willis
Illustrator: Kerrie Hess
Production: Rachel Burgess

This book reports information and opinions which may be of general
interest to the reader. It is advisory only and is not intended to serve as
a substitution for a consultation with a dermatologist, beauty therapist
or physician. Neither the author nor the publisher can accept
responsibility for any accident, injury or damage that results from using
the ideas, information or advice offered in this book.

The application and quality of beauty products, treatments, herbal
preparations and essential oils is beyond the control of the above
parties who cannot be held responsible for any problems resulting from
their use. Always follow the manufacturer's instructions. Do not use
herbal preparations or essential oils without prior consultation with a
qualified practitioner or medical doctor, if you are pregnant, taking any
form of medication or if you suffer from oversensitive skin.

# CONTENTS

# INTRODUCTION

**Did you know that ketchup can help correct green tinges in blonde hair, that sun damage makes pores larger or that using a cool, bright lipstick colour will make your teeth look whiter?**

Here we've gathered together 1001 little beauty tricks and tips to help you get gorgeous from head to toe. Read through the categories that interest you or dip in and out to get quick, succinct advice for any beauty problem you face. From acne outbreaks to untidy eyebrows, from split ends to cellulite, you will find new techniques and solutions to help you improve the appearance and health of your body and let you put your best face forward every day.

# Top ten little beauty miracles

## 33
**KNOW YOUR NASTIES**
(see Cosmeceuticals & miracle ingredients, page 16)

## 165
**CHOOSE A VERSATILE PRODUCT**
(see Base-ic rights, page 44)

## 200
**DIVIDE BY FOUR**
(see Brows, page 51)

**594**
WEAR IT NAKED
(see Fragrance, page 129)

**701**
FILE FIRST
(see Nails, page 151)

**811**
BREATHE YOURSELF
BEAUTIFUL
(see Inner beauty,
page 174)

**251**
DON'T GO TOO LIGHT
(see Conceal it, page 58)

**282**
BE ALL WHITE
(see Eyeliner, page 64)

**342**
DO 3-D LIPS
(see Lips, page 75)

**388**
CURL AWAY
(see Mascara, page 81)

# SKINCARE

# anti-ageing

**1 SAFEGUARD SENIOR SKIN**

The skin on your face is the thinnest on the body and the older the skin, the thinner and drier it can be. It will need extra protection and moisture, especially in the harsh winter months, so moisturize frequently and avoid harsh toners.

**2 BE ALERT TO BETACAROTENE**

Betacarotene, a powerful natural anti-ageing antioxidant, is a pigment in yellow and red fresh foods that the body converts to vitamin A to generate new cells. Get your dose from apricots, peaches, nectarines, sweet potatoes, carrots and leafy greens.

**3 SEEK OUT SELENIUM**

Fish, red meat, chicken, grains and eggs contain selenium, an antioxidant which works with vitamin E against pollutants to combat skin ageing and cancer. Healthy sources include oil-rich nuts, seeds and avocados.

## 4 GET AN EARLY START

It's best to start using anti-ageing creams in your thirties and forties to get maximum effects. Before that, their richness will be too heavy for younger skins.

## 5 DON'T MAKE THE FACE

Making faces and adopting signature facial expressions creates folds and wrinkles between the brows and eyes. Simply being aware of your facial expressions (particularly in the sun) will stop them appearing in the first place.

## 6 SMOOTH AWAY FINE LINES

To prevent ageing and ensure the delicate skin around your eyes stays taut, apply an eye cream above and below the eye area morning and night after the age of 25.

## 7 COOK UP A WRINKLE-FREE SKIN

If you want skin as smooth as a tomato, eat one. Tomatoes contain lycopene, a skin-friendly antioxidant that is also thought to reduce cancer risk. Cooking tomatoes makes lycopene more available.

## 8 LOOK GREAT WITH GRAPES

Resveratrol, a polyphenol found in red grapes and an antioxidant and anti-cancer agent, helps mop up the damage caused by sun and pollution exposure, allowing the skin to help heal itself following damage. In addition to eating grapes, look for vinotherapy salon treatments and products that claim to harvest this ingredient.

## 9 STAY OUT OF THE SUN

Ninety per cent of problems associated with ageing are the result of too much sun exposure, so the best thing you can do to help your skin stay young is avoid the sun.

## 10 GET YOUR BEAUTY SLEEP

Sleep is one of the best ways to reduce the signs of ageing, by allowing skin to replenish overnight. If you can't sleep, make sure your room isn't too hot – the deepest sleep occurs if your atmosphere is 18–24°C (64–75°F).

## 11 PICK UP PYCNOGENOL

Pycnogenol is an antioxidant found in pine bark that contains vitamins A, C and E as well as its own age-busters. It is claimed to reverse and prevent wrinkles, so look out for it on products' ingredient lists for an anti-ageing boost.

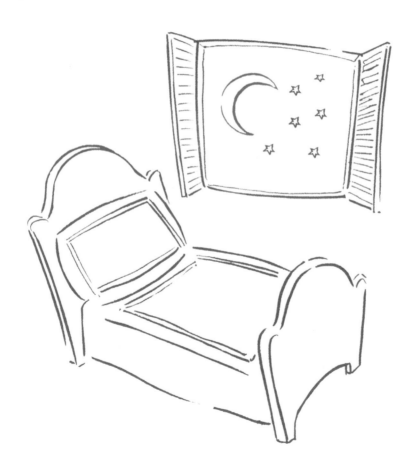

## 12 GIVE UP SMOKING

In smokers, skin looks sallow as a result of poor circulation and the action of drawing on the cigarette causes lines to be etched around the mouth. To reduce these signs of ageing, give up smoking if you're still doing it, and avoid smoky environments.

## 13 BE FRANK ABOUT AGEING

Frankincense is thought to have some anti-ageing effects by plumping up the skin and forming a protective barrier against further damage and stress. Find it in specialist creams and salon treatments.

## 14 GO KOJIC FOR AGE SPOTS

Treat skin discolouration, such as freckles and age spots, with Kojic acid, discovered in Japan in 1989 and derived from fungi. It is gentle on the skin and rebalances discoloured skin by penetrating upper skin layers to inhibit uneven pigment formation. Results can be seen after four to six weeks. Vitamin A and mulberry extract are other ingredients that have pigment-levelling properties.

## 15 GET LIPPY

For an anti-ageing make-up effect, keep the eyes bare and wear a strong colour on the lips. This will draw attention away from lines and wrinkles around the eyes and emphasize the shape of lips and lower jaw, giving a more youthful appearance.

## 16 DRINK IT IN

Overall skin health depends on proper hydration, as the skin is the first organ to become dehydrated if you don't drink enough, causing sagging and lines. The optimum amount is 2.5 litres (5 pints) a day.

# cleansing & care

## 17 BEWARE OF OVERCLEANSING

Overcleansing is a major cause of sensitive skin, as it strips the skin's underlayers of its natural protective properties. Make sure you use a cleanser that's right for your skin type and don't overdo it.

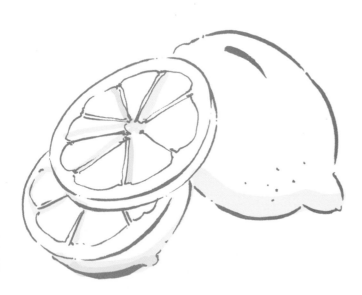

## 18 GIVE IT A REST

Moisturizer seals in more than moisture – it stops oil escaping from the skin and can cause spots in those prone to breakouts. Occasionally give yourself a break from night-time creams to allow your skin to breathe and regulate itself normally.

## 19 STEAM AWAY IMPURITIES

For a quick, deep cleanse, pour boiling water into a bowl with lemon juice and rose petals and hold your face over the bowl, covering your head with a towel. The steam will invigorate you, aid in respiration, and help loosen blackheads. Cleanse afterwards and follow with a cool-water rinse to close pores.

## 20 GO LARGE

Remember that for cleansing, moisturizing and facial skincare purposes, your face is the area between your hairline and your collarbone – don't neglect that neck skin. Not only is the skin soft and delicate, it is also very close to underlying structures like the thyroid and voice box. Gentle is best.

## 21 TIP OF THE DAY

When cleansing, many people forget the tip of their nose, which can then become oily or greasy. Use small circular movements to make sure you get your whole nose clean!

## 22 SLEEP CLEAN

It's an old adage, but never go to bed with your make-up on. It prevents the skin from shedding and breathing and may cause blemishes and/or blackheads to appear.

## 23 SPECIALIZE FOR EYES

For fast removal, use a good eye make-up remover rather than a cleanser. It has oils that dissolve make-up better and faster than regular cleanser or toner. Then wash as usual.

## 24 ASSESS TO CLEANSE BEST

Your first step in the morning should be to take a good look in the mirror. Note any dry patches on the cheeks or oiliness in the T-zone. Hormones, seasons, environment and diet can all impact on your skin and will be evident – you can then adjust your regime accordingly.

## 25 KEEP YOUR HAIR OFF THE SKIN

Keep hair clean and off the face to avoid making skin greasy, especially overnight when it can rub against skin as you sleep and cause spots and blemishes to appear.

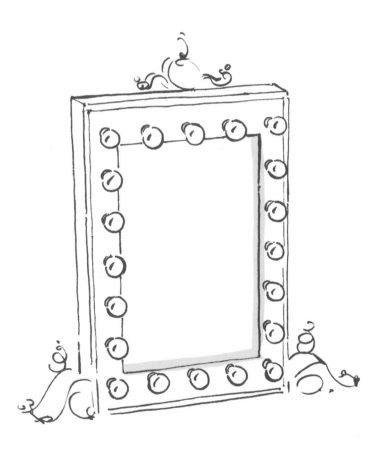

## 26 PLEASE WASH YOUR HANDS

Make sure your hands are clean before you touch your face. When applying the foundation, use a sponge or brush to give a velvety look.

## 27 CLEANSE BEFORE YOU COLOUR

Before applying your make-up in the morning, make sure you thoroughly cleanse your face and apply moisturizer to even out the skin.

# cosmeceuticals & miracle ingredients

## 28 GET SMOOTH WITH SOY

Soy proteins can help make skin temporarily smoother by improving firmness and elasticity if applied regularly. Look for them as ingredients in new hi-tech face creams.

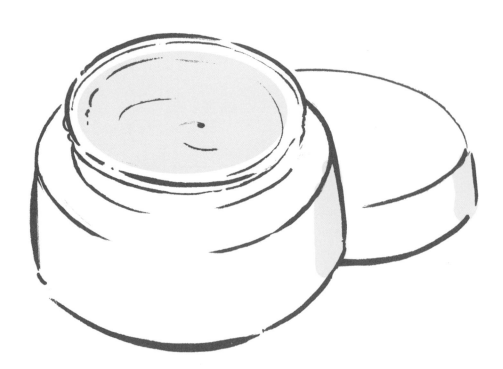

## 29 PAPAYA FOR PAPAIN ENZYME

Papaya contains the papain enzyme, a natural, nonabrasive botanical that dissolves dead skin cells, which makes it a great ingredient for face masks and exfoliators. It deep cleanses without stripping, leaving dull skin smoother and more refined.

## 30 QUEUE UP FOR CO-Q10

Co-enzyme Q10 is a natural antioxidant found in every cell of the body that helps fight bacteria and free radicals and allows cells to grow and repair. Incorporated in anti-wrinkle creams, the synthetic version can reduce lines and deter new ones.

## 31 GO MAD FOR MANGOSTIN

If you suffer from redness, blotchiness and broken capillaries on the skin, look for Mangostin in your face cream. An extract from the mangosteen fruit, Mangostin has been shown to help reduce red patches, dark spots and other circulation-related troubles, particularly when combined with antioxidant vitamins A, C and E.

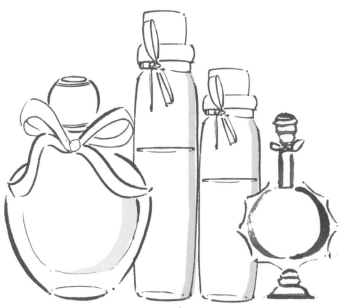

## 32 COTTON RICH

Cotton is the latest natural ingredient to hit the headlines – especially for dry skins. The structure of cottonseed oils can help skin lock away moisture and stay hydrated for longer.

## 33 KNOW YOUR NASTIES

If you're worried about chemicals and toxins in products, the main ones to steer clear of on ingredients lists are: propylene glycol (used in antifreeze), isopropyl alcohol, methylisothiazolinone, sodium lauryl sulphate (used in engine degreaser), formaldehyde, stearalkonium chloride, DEA (diethanolanine) and TEA (triethanolinine).

## 34 C THE DIFFERENCE

Vitamin C (ascorbic acid) has a brightening effect on skin as it helps boost circulation and collagen production, which means skin looks and feels firmer and smoother as a result. It is essential to the formation of collagen. Vitamin C is found in high levels in citrus fruits, berries and kiwi, but also in serums, creams and other beauty products.

## 35 CUCUMBER AND THYME

Cucumber and thyme contain anti-inflammatory and antiseptic properties to soothe red, irritated skin, and are thought to be especially powerful when used in combination with each other, as they exert stronger effects.

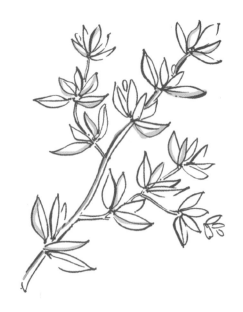

## 36 GET HELP FROM AHA

Alpha-hydroxy acids (AHAs), found in many anti-ageing products, are organic chemicals derived from fruit-bearing plants, hence often called 'fruit acids'. Thought to help generate new collagen, making skin firmer and plumper, they also dissolve the 'glue' that binds dead cells, allowing the old ones to be washed or cleansed away and revealing younger cells.

## 37 WEAR A MICRO MINERAL

Micronized titanium and zinc oxide mineral make-up provide sun protection and minimize itching and burning. Due to the fact that these powders are composed completely of micronized rock, they cannot grow bacteria, which makes them safe for use on sensitive and healing skin.

## 38 LIGHTEN UP WITH LIQUORICE

Liquorice extract has been shown to have an evening and lightening effect on skin that will help fade age and sun spots if used over a few months. Many anti-ageing creams now contain it.

## 39 TAKE UP TOCOPHEROL

The ingredient alpha-tocopherol, found in face creams and sunscreens, is thought to optimize protection against damaging UVA and UVB rays, help prevent premature signs of ageing and stimulate collagen production to make the skin look younger.

## 40 AXE WRINKLES WITH ASTAXANTHIN

Astaxanthin is a carotenoid pigment and powerful 'super' antioxidant. Derived from natural oils, it is thought to have regenerating and rejuvenating effects on the skin, is an anti-inflammatory, plumps up skin and reduces the appearance of blemishes and wrinkles. It offers superb protection against environment damage.

## 41 SHARK IT UP

Look for anti-ageing creams with shark cartilage included. The ingredient stimulates the natural production of collagen and elastin in the skin, making it look and feel younger, firmer and plumper. It is an anti-inflammatory and anti-angiogenic.

## 42 SILICA SOLUTIONS

Concentrated organic silica builds up keratin in hair and nails by providing the basic building blocks for new keratin to be formed. These products are often derived from sea shells, which also contain other marine boosters.

## 43 MEASURE THE MARIGOLDS

Marigold – mainly listed on cosmetics packages as calendula – is an excellent choice for calming sore, swollen skin and contains natural anti-inflammatory properties which make it great for sensitive skins.

## 44 ZINC IT UP

When it comes to skin-boosting minerals, zinc is the number one choice as it has a direct effect on the regeneration of skin from the inside out, which can not only help problem and ageing skins but will also give your skin a healthy glow and banish dullness.

## 45 PLANT PROTEINS

Some plant proteins have been shown to be almost as effective over short periods as salon treatments for smoothing skin and reducing wrinkles.

## 46 REPAIR TISSUES WITH B5

Vitamin B5 is known to assist with tissue repair, which can help the skin to feel smoother and younger because it repairs problems in the deeper layers and prevents blemishes and fine lines.

## 47 SAY YES TO SAFFLOWER

Increasingly, cosmetic companies are waking up to the benefits of safflower oil to create and purify emulsions. The product increases the skin's absorption of oils without making it oily, so is a great choice for anti-ageing creams.

## 48 LOOK YOUNGER WITH MESOTHERAPY

Mesotherapy, in which vitamins, minerals and antioxidants are injected into the middle layer of the skin, is said to improve skin quality and vitality by replenishing the skin with essential vitamins that occur naturally within the cells. The vitamins A, E, C, D and B create firmness, clarity and smoothness in the skin.

## 49 REGENERATE WITH RETINOID

Retinoid is a vitamin A compound, available through pharmacies in the prescription Retin-A and in cosmeceuticals as retinol, which can help reduce fine lines and wrinkles by regenerating skin in the lower layers, sloughing off the upper layers and by stimulating collagen and elastin.

## 50 REDUCE REDNESS WITH BHAS

BHAs, beta-hydroxy acids that include salicylic acid, help shed excess skin cells with their chemical sloughing effect and they are also anti-inflammatories, which make skin appear less red and inflamed, and reduce puffiness. Gentler than AHAs, they can also treat acne.

## 51 VITAMIN COCKTAILS

BioVityl and VitaNiacin technology is the newest way to give skin a vitamin boost, by combining vitamins the skin needs in one formula. The combination of vitamins cleverly increases absorption and makes the creams work better.

## 52 THINK ZINC

Zinc sulphate products like Cellex-C are naturally derived from plants and sometimes shellfish and have been claimed to have anti-ageing effects by smoothing the skin and protecting it from dehydration. It can help clear complexions prone to blemishes and can improve colour, tone and texture.

## 53 HYDROQUINONE FOR HYPERPIGMENTATION

Hydroquinone is a chemical ingredient in skin creams (and can appear under a wide range of brand names), which eases the appearance of patchy skin caused by hyperpigmentation. It is often delivered in a hyalauronic acid base to smooth the texture of skin further.

## 54 FADE AWAY FRECKLES

Kojic acid and arbutin are natural alternatives to hydroquinone (see above), which work synergistically to help break up hyperpigmentation in the skin's layers by levelling out melanin levels. They have been used successfully for fading age spots, freckles and sun spots.

## 55 MAKE MINE A MAGNESIUM

Magnesium has been shown to reduce the appearance of fine lines and wrinkles in skin by helping to tighten the surface of the skin and boost the production of new skin cells. It is often found as an ingredient in age-defying polishers.

## 56 SAY HELLO TO HYALAURONIC ACID

Hyalauronic acid is a powerful ingredient that occurs naturally within our cells and contributes to the structural support of the skin if it soaks into the lower layers. Best used as a face mask or leave-on cream.

## 57 LOOK FOR LIPOLIC

Alpha-lipolic acid (not to be confused with alpha-hydroxy acid) is nature's most powerful anti-inflammatory and anti-oxidant treatment, which is many times more powerful than vitamins alone for skin healing and hydration.

## 58 LATCH ONTO LACTIC ACID

Lactic acid is a wonderful ingredient for extra moisturization because it helps the skin hold onto the moisture that's being added through creams and lotions. It's especially useful in anti-wrinkle and anti-ageing products.

## 59 GIVE SKIN A FEAST

Skin is the last organ to get the benefits of the good things you eat, so often there's precious little nourishment left, even if your diet is fantastic. Choose face treatments high in essential minerals such as calcium, magnesium and zinc to give it a boost.

## 60 ANTI-STRETCH STRIVECTIN

StriVectin is a formulation in face and body creams, which includes skin-firming agents, elasticizers and skin hydrators, that has been shown to lead to visible stretchmark and wrinkle reduction.

## 61 C FOR YOURSELF

Vitamin C is a natural skin protector, necessary for the formation of collagen. As an antioxidant it destroys harmful free-radicals in the body caused by pollution, stress and bad diet. Free radicals attack the skin, causing premature ageing, so vitamin C in creams and diet is a must.

## 62 BOOST OILS NATURALLY

One of the major skin health-boosting ingredients in creams and lotions is essential fatty acids, which can plump the skin and help stop it drying out with their non-greasy, oil-producing texture.

## 63 HANDS OFF OILY SKIN

Touching, stroking and facial massage stimulates the skin's oil glands to produce more sebum, which is the last thing oily skin needs. So, if you want to dry it out, keep your hands off your face.

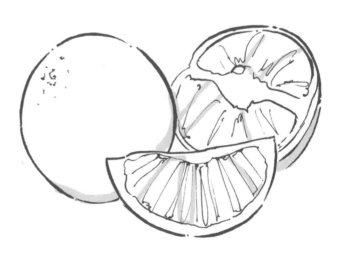

# creams & serums

## 64 EXTREME CREAMS

Hydroquinone is a common ingredient in skin-bleaching creams, but as it works by killing off the top layers of skin cells, some people find it makes their skin look older and causes sensitivity. Use with care.

## 65 USE LESS THAN YOU THINK

Don't slather on more product in the belief that it will work better. Many good products are highly concentrated and only designed to be used in very small amounts.

## 66 DAY AND NIGHT

Always use separate day and night creams. The day creams are designed to absorb into the skin quickly and not interfere with make-up application whereas night creams are more emollient and designed for bare skin.

## 67 GLOW WITH SERUM

Unlike moisturizers, serums – either in bottle form or as ampoules – have an oily rather than absorbent texture and impart a glow to the skin that improves the visual appearance. They can be used as a quick pick-me-up to give an instant richness to skin's texture.

## 68 MOISTURIZE ONE AT A TIME

It's a common mistake to buy three or four similar products, open them all and alternate using them. But if you do this, the chances are that you won't use them all before their use-by date and they'll end up going off or being ineffective.

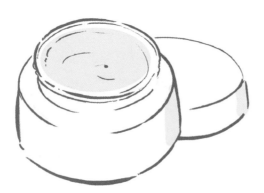

## 68 NIGHT-TIME BEAUTY

Beauty sleep is not a myth. While you sleep, your skin regenerates itself, which is why night creams are such a good idea for moisture. Make sure you go to bed hydrated so the skin gets a chance to heal itself.

## 70 FIRM AND MOISTURIZE

For very dry or mature skin, a firming serum or treatment applied underneath a moisturizer gives an added boost.

## 71 TREAT COMBINED AREAS

A one-product moisturizer that contains AHAs should treat and normalize both dry and oily areas equally. There are also cleansers available with ingredients that leave dry areas moisturized and oily areas cleared of sebum.

## 72 PROTECT WITH UV

Always use a moisturizer with an SPF 15 to protect from sun damage. With modern formulations there is no need to apply both a sunscreen and a moisturizer.

## 73 DO IT DAILY WITH LIGHT MOISTURIZING

Every skin type needs a daily moisturizer, so know the one suitable for you. Lightweight gels and simple moisturizers are good for young and sensitive skins.

## 74 SERUMS ARE SERIOUSLY GOOD

Serums are pumps or vials of potent anti-ageing agents such as antioxidants and AHAs. Some are formulated for daily use under a moisturizer while others are for short-term or overnight use.

## 75 NIGHT-TIME TREATS

Choose products especially for overnight use – these are packed with vitamins and usually have a specific delivery system that enables the skin to maximize the extra regeneration of cells that occurs during the night.

## 76 DO IT SENSITIVELY

If you have easily reactive or sensitive skin, stick to simple, pure products without a cocktail of anti-ageing or AHA ingredients. These will simply replenish the natural moisture without triggering a problem.

## 77 USE IT OR LOSE IT

When putting on a face cream, scrub or mask instead of wiping or washing off what's left, use it up on the backs of hands and fingers to keep them looking younger and well-conditioned for longer.

## 78 AVOID REACTIVE SKIN

Use a cream with a mild hydrocortisone included for problem skin that is prone to rashes and redness. The anti-inflammatory products will help your skin maintain a healthy profile.

# exfoliators & scrubs

## 79 EXFOLIATE FOR EXCEPTIONAL SKIN

If left on the body, dead skin cells flake, dry and peel quickly, so the best way to keep skin looking smooth, vital and evenly coloured is to scrub away those dead cells with a shower scrub.

## 80 MAKE YOUR OWN

For a super-smoothing skin exfoliant, massage a handful of Epsom salts with a tablespoon of olive oil over wet skin to cleanse, exfoliate and soften the rough spots. Rinse off well for a polished finish.

## 81 BE AVOCADO FAIR

For a natural exfoliant, grate an avocado stone with a small grater and add it to a little yogurt, cream or avocado flesh. Use the mixture to polish the skin, then rinse off.

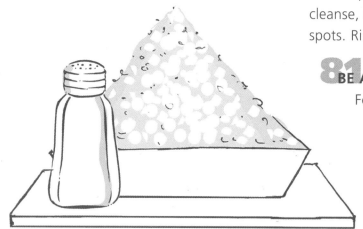

## 82 BRUSH AND GO

If your lips are seriously dry or flaky, apply a little lip balm and brush them with a soft, dry toothbrush to boost circulation and remove all the dead skin cells while working the moisturizer into the deeper levels of your skin.

## 83 TINGLE AWAY

Generally, tingling after exfoliation means you've used too harsh a product, but it is natural to tingle for up to 15 minutes after using alpha- or beta-hydroxy acids to exfoliate because of their chemical effect.

## 84 EXFOLIATE WITH CARE

Don't be tempted to rub too hard or use a too-grainy exfoliant on your face. Instead, choose small-grained products and keep it to once a week. If your skin looks red or patchy, you've gone too far.

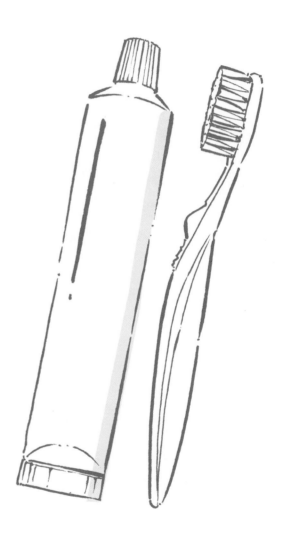

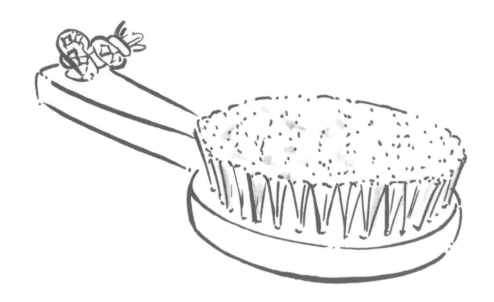

## 85 SHIELD IN THE SUN

Newly exfoliated skin is more prone to sun damage, so apply a sun block after exfoliating if you're going to be exposed.

## 86 RUB AWAY ROUGH ELBOWS

If your elbows are very dry, put a small amount of foot exfoliator in the palm of your hand and rub in circular motions. This will be too harsh for the skin of your arms, but works a treat to lift off excess elbow skin.

## 87 STAY NATURAL WITH SALT

Salt is nature's own favourite exfoliator. Not only do the sharp grains help you exfoliate skin gently and without trauma, the natural healing and antiseptic qualities help your skin stay smooth, supple and problem free.

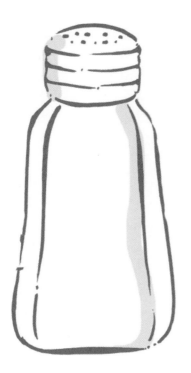

## 88 FACE FACTS WEEKLY

On your face, you should exfoliate once a week to remove dead skin cells. This will not only make your skin look fresher and more radiant, but also helps your products penetrate deeper into the epidermis, making them more effective.

## 89 STOP INGROWERS

Regular exfoliation has been shown to help prevent ingrown hairs and promote smoother skin as the skin 'gets used' to regenerating itself in response to the upper layers being removed efficiently.

## 90 DON'T MIX FACE AND BODY

Don't be tempted to use body exfoliators on facial skin, because products designed for the body are likely to be harsher and could be too abrasive for your face, resulting in irritation.

## 91 DON'T FORGET BUTTOCKS

It might not be the first thing people see about you, but don't neglect the skin of your buttocks, which can be prone to pimples and cellulite, if left untended. Use a bath mitt or puff to gently exfoliate in the bath or shower.

## 92 MOISTURIZE ALL THE WAY

If you exfoliate regularly, you should always use moisturizer on your face because the regular exfoliation could lead to skin drying up more easily as a result of having fewer layers. You should use it even on the days you're not exfoliating for best results.

## 93 GO GENTLY

Overly vigorous exfoliating can break the tiny blood vessels under your skin, causing thread veins and redness to appear, especially on the delicate skin around the cheeks, eyes and neck. Be gentle and avoid exfoliators with natural grains, which are more abrasive than synthetics.

## 94 VOTE VOLCANIC

Some exfoliating cleansers contain as much as 25 per cent ground volcanic rock. These are good for oily skin because they dry up oil without stripping too much out of the skin and causing a rebound effect.

## 95 EXFOLIATE BUMPS

It's not just your face that needs exfoliating – skin bumps on legs can occur as a result of ingrown hairs. To avoid them, exfoliate legs regularly with a grainy scrub in the shower, then apply moisturizer.

## 96 GIVE NATURE A HAND

Every 24 hours, we lose an astounding 10 billion cells from the skin's surface, though as we age our skin cells take longer to renew. Exfoliating once a week or more helps boost this natural process, preventing blemishes and dull skin caused by the build-up of dead skin cells and revealing a clearer complexion.

# skin problems

### 97 POLLUTION PROTECTION

Battle against polluted urban environments by using an SPF foundation or day cream specifically formulated to screen out the sun naturally with titanium dioxide, rather than one that contains chemicals, which will contribute to the overload of toxins and environmental chemicals.

### 98 STAY COOL TO CURE CAPILLARIES

For the ultimate in smooth, blemish-free skin, try to stay cool. Overheating can cause damage to fine capillaries in the cheeks and nose, which may contribute to and worsen redness and blotchiness.

### 99 AVOID BLEACH FOR VITILIGO

Repigmentation programmes involving steroid creams, UV light and surgery can help address the white patches of vitiligo, but must be administered by a professional. Bleaching agents have side effects and are not the best option for dark skins.

### 100 HELP FOR PSORIASIS

Traditionally treated with coal-tar and emollients, new creams containing vitamins D3 and A have proved beneficial. Dithranol, derived from the araroba tree, can be used for isolated incidences and has been proven to kill off the rapidly reproducing cells that cause the problem.

### 101 EASE ECZEMA

The red, blistering itchy skin of eczema can be treated with a triceram cream, a nonsteroid with a ceramide base that helps the skin to repair. Balloon vine extract is an anti-inflammatory that can also help and is available in gel form.

### 102 SENSE YOUR SENSITIVITY

If your skin is reactive, try to find out the triggers, whether they are environmental, nutritional or from using certain skincare products. Bolster your skin's barrier with a moisturizer for sensitive skin and protect it from extremes of weather. Dehydrated skin is more susceptible to infections, immune disorders and sun damage.

### 103 DRIER THAN DUST

For skin tightness, cracking and flaking, choose a cream cleanser rather than a soap-based one and never use drying toners.

### 104 ARREST PREMATURE AGEING

Rescue ageing skin by being scrupulous about using a sunscreen daily, keep out of the sun in summer and rescue early fine lines with intensive serums and brightening AHAs. You must use an SPF15 in combination with acids such as AHA and BHA.

### 105 NO ROSÉ FOR ROSACEA

If you suffer rosacea, avoid alcohol as this increases blood flow to the face, which can cause an increase in redness. It also dehydrates, which may make skin appear dryer.

### 106 USE LESS ON ECZEMA

When it comes to covering sensitive skin conditions such as eczema, less is definitely more. Use too much powder or base and you risk highlighting the dryness and uneven texture.

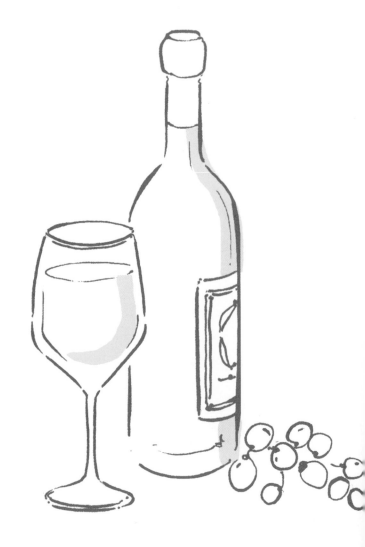

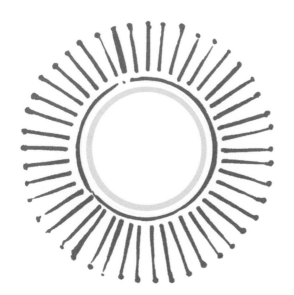

## 107 FOR SMALL PORES, STAY OUT OF THE SUN

Sun damage – both long-term and short-term – makes pores appear larger because the sun's UV rays break down collagen, making the tissues around your pores weaker and causing the epidermis to thicken. The effects can be permanent.

## 108 KEEP CLEAN TO ARREST ACNE SPREAD

After using brushes or concealer sticks to cover up blemishes or spots, always wash them well to avoid re-infection when you use them again. Or use cotton buds, which are disposable. Also keep your hands away from your face and pay particular attention to habits like rubbing the temples or around the mouth, which you may do subconsciously.

## 109 SPICE ISN'T NICE

Rosacea can be exacerbated by spicy foods containing chilli and mustard as well as hot drinks, which cause an increase in circulation and can make redness worse, as well as causing skin to feel hot and uncomfortable.

## 110 HARSH PRODUCTS CAN HARM

If you suffer from rosacea, you should at all times avoid astringents and harsh soaps because not only can they make the symptoms worse, they also dry out skin, making it harder to treat and cover.

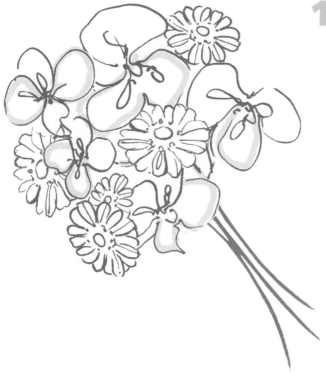

## 111 IT'S HIP TO BE ROSE

For dry skin, choose products containing extract of rosehip. This ingredient contains high levels of omega-3 and omega-6 oils, which are nourishing for the skin. It also acts as an anti-inflammatory, which will soothe problem areas.

## 112 STOP ACNE ADVANCEMENT

If you suffer from recurring boils and spots, book an appointment with a private dermatologist immediately – they will be able to prescribe a specific course of action that neither yourself, your pharmacist nor your normal GP has the expertise to diagnose. Allowing the problem to linger means months without a solution.

## 113 STAY COOL TO CONTROL ECZEMA

Eczema symptoms can be exacerbated by extremes of temperature and respond particularly badly to overheating. Make sure you stay cool by seeking shade and choosing natural fabrics. Changing your laundry detergent may also help.

## 114 UNPLUG BLACKHEADS

One of the most effective ways to rid yourself of blackheads without damaging or bruising your skin is with pore-cleaning strips, available over the counter from most pharmacies. Because the skin isn't squeezed with this technique, it is not at risk from further infection.

## 115 WASH WHITEHEADS AWAY

Keep whiteheads at bay on spot-prone skin by washing greasy areas only with a mild cleanser that contains benzoyl peroxide and glycolic acids, which in combination have been shown to reduce the severity of pimples.

## 116 PEEL OFF THE LAYERS

You can now get similar results at home as you would from a medically administered chemical peel because of advances in technology. Over-the-counter 'peel' kits contain chemicals such as glycolic acid that dissolve the top layers of skin, lifting them off to reveal a brighter complexion. They usually have a two- or three-part process: the acid solution, an agent to calm the skin and stop the action and a moisturizer.

## 117 TREAT SPOTS WITH FACIALS

Regular professionally administered facials can help prevent spots because they keep your pores cleaner than you can at home. They'll also help facial muscles relax and keep your skin hydrated and plump.

## 117 PORES FOR THOUGHT

The best way to keep pores looking smaller and tighter is to keep them clean, washing your face twice a day – morning and evening – for best results with a mild cleanser.

## 118 PEROXIDE FOR PIMPLES

If you're prone to spotty breakouts, use a benzoyl peroxide solution on the affected area, which will dry out the area of oil and which also has antibacterial properties, which can help stop spots appearing.

## 119 WORK AWAY WHITEHEADS

If you suffer whiteheads, try applying a gel or cream containing salicylic acid to the pimple, a drying and toning agent which may help you to unplug the pores and prevent further outbreaks.

## 120 TRY SHORT-TERM STEROIDS

Topical steroids can be used on a short-term basis to help reduce the symptoms of rosacea, but long term use may actually make it worse because it thins the skin and can cause other problems.

## 121 STEM THE ERUPTION

Cystic acne has the potential to leave deep scars so spots should never be squeezed. If it's an open pimple, apply an acne-drying gel or lotion and let it run its course. If you have frequent outbreaks, see a dermatologist.

## 122 HEAT IT UP

If you have to squeeze blackheads, apply a warm-to-hot flannel first to soften, then wrap a tissue around your fingers and gently squeeze. Never squeeze facial skin hard enough to leave an imprint.

## 123 HIDE BEHIND THE SCREEN

If you notice pigment patches on your cheeks or forehead, wear high-protection sunscreen at all times to minimize further damage and ensure your skin stays as even as possible.

## 124 CLARIFY WITH CLAY

If you suffer from red, inflamed blemishes, use a clay-based mask or drying lotion to help draw out any impurities and reduce swelling. Apply only to the affected area if the rest of your skin is dry.

## 126 BOTTLE THE MOTTLE

If you have mottled skin or patchy colouring, many heavy, penetrating moisturizers can help disguise and correct uneven pigmentation, giving the complexion a smoother, more even appearance. Opt for one with built-in sunscreen to prevent further problems.

## 127 STEAM IT AWAY

It's almost impossible to prevent blackheads, but steam can help minimize them. Once a week, steam your face to soften the oils that clog the pores and follow with a deep-cleansing clay skin mask, rinsing thoroughly with warm water to clear the skin.

## 128 PREVENT SPREAD

If you're worried about infection from acne eruptions spreading to other parts of your face, use a topical antibiotic, which will help to contain the infection. Never squeeze, as it could make the pore swell further and look worse, and avoid metal extractor tools which can damage surrounding tissue.

## 129 MAKE IT BRIEF

If you suffer from dry skin, try not to spend too long in the bath or shower, and avoid over-washing your face. The constant wetting and drying serves to dehydrate your skin.

## 130 KEEP IT SIMPLE

If you suffer from irregular pigmentation, don't overcomplicate your skincare. Avoid harsh sponges and exfoliating rubs, and don't use toner, which can exacerbate pigment differences.

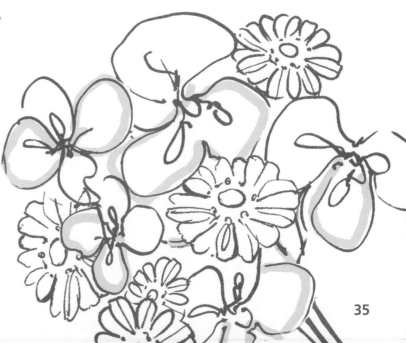

## 131 PIGMENT SKIN ALERT

If you are pregnant or suffer irregular skin pigmentation, avoid bergamot essential oil as this can cause uneven skin colour to become worse. Some concentrations are photo-toxic, and can accelerate pigmentation by making skin more sensitive to sunlight. Avoid exposure to the sun, sun lamps or tanning booths if using the oil.

## 132 HOLD THE SCRUB

Beware of over-exfoliating spotty or oily areas of the skin. On problem skin, exfoliation can cause excess oils to be released, making the problem worse, and it can cause acne to spread to uninfected areas. Instead, use gentle polishers to treat the oily areas only.

## 133 NO PICKING

Try to avoid picking or touching spots. Not only will grease and grime from your fingers be spread onto your skin, but picking can also cause scarring and pigmentation marks as well as increasing infection risk.

## 134 FACIAL HARMONY

To improve red, itchy or allergic skins, visit a salon for a specific ultra-sensitive skin treatment. If plant-based products like arnica and cypress nut are used, they will reduce swelling and redness.

## 135 SCENT SENSITIVITY

Instead of using a scented sunscreen on sensitive skins, opt for an unscented alternative that contains organic, plant-based ingredients, such as aloe vera, jojoba, avocado and camomile.

# toners

## 136 AVOID THE TINGLE

In general, products that make your skin tingle are too harsh – tingling in response to toners or cleansers is your skin's way of telling you to go for something weaker. Try toners that are designed for sensitive skin – look for those based on rosewater instead of witch hazel or alcohol.

## 137 NORMAL WISDOM

If you have normal skin, make sure you choose a light moisturizer, especially one that is formulated as a lotion or gel. Too-rich moisturizers can trigger spots and blemishes by blocking pores.

## 138 BE A T-ZONE SMOOTHIE

If you have combination skin, treat the different areas of your face independently – exfoliate the T-zone area, but leave cheeks alone, and when moisturizing concentrate on cheeks and neck, leaving only a light layer on the T-zone.

## 139 POUR COLD WATER ON IT

For a quick tone and boost for tired, dull skin, splash your face in cold water to bring fresh blood to the surface, stimulating circulation and giving you a healthy glow.

## 140 WITCHES' BREW

If you run out of toner, witch hazel mixed with a little water is a natural alternative, but be careful on older skins which can dry excessively if the mix is too concentrated.

## 141 BE ALCOHOL-FREE

Alcohol-based toners and cleansers are the enemy of dry skin, as they strip the skin dry of moisture and can cause problems with skin firmness and blemishes. If you suffer from dry skin, avoid products with alcohol and use a moisturizer more than once a day to keep skin plump and hydrated.

## 142 STOP THE BATH SOAP

Whatever your skin type, avoid using even mild bath soap on the sensitive skin of your face, neck and behind the ears, as this can leave skin feeling tight and drained at best, and can cause redness and rashes to develop. Choose a cleanser that is specially formulated for your face.

## 143 DON'T BE A WASHOUT

If you have oily skin, the worst thing you can do is overwash or use a harsh cleanser, as these will actually encourage more production of oils in the skin and could make you spottier. Avoid products that strip the skin and opt for lotions rather than heavy creams.

# wrinkle-busters

## 144 SILK SIREN

For the smoothest facial skin, copy the Egyptian queens and insist on a silk or satin pillow, which will smooth out facial wrinkles while you sleep and ensure you wake up looking your best.

## 145 KNOW YOUR WRINKLES

There are four different types of wrinkles – fine, deep, static and dynamic. Fine wrinkles, around the eyes, occur gradually due to the breakdown of collagen and elastin; deeper ones like forehead lines start in the muscles below the surface; dynamic lines are those seen only when your face moves; and static wrinkles are seen all the time.

## 146 WALK WRINKLES AWAY

Walking delivers oxygen to the complexion, gets blood flowing and reduces tension-related wrinkles because it releases feel-good chemicals in the body, which reduce stress and boost relaxation.

## 147 DON'T CONFUSE WRINKLES WITH DRYNESS

Dry skin can look more wrinkled, but actual wrinkles are not due to dry skin: they are due to damage to the skin's underlayers from ageing, sun exposure and smoking, as well as other pollutants. Moisturize and drink plenty of water to avoid dehydration.

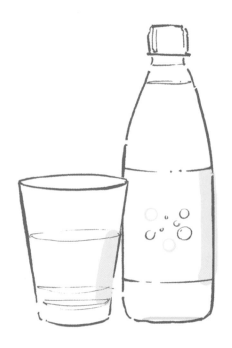

## 147 REPAIR YOUR SKIN

Vitamin A can help diminish wrinkle depth,
as its light inflammatory action 'puffs
up' the skin so wrinkles look less
deep. Find it in anti-wrinkle
creams or add it to your diet
by eating lots of fruit and
vegetables.

## 148 WHITE AND GREEN TEA

Green and white tea can
help delay collagen ageing
and weakening, which
has been shown to
be a premier cause
of wrinkles. Many face
creams use green and
white tea, not only for
their anti-oxidant properties
but also because white tea is
shown to limit DNA damage in sun-
exposed skin. White tea promotes new cell
growth and strengthens the skin.

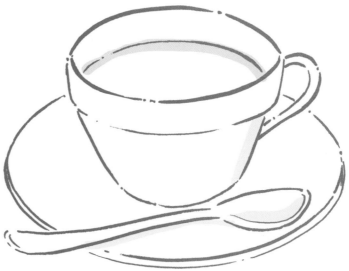

## 150 WEIGHT ON FOR A SMOOTH FACE

Rapid weight loss can cause wrinkles by reducing the volume of fat cells that cushion the face. This not only makes you look gaunt, but can cause the skin to sag.

## 151 KEEP YOUR BROWLINE FREE

Squinting is a common cause of wrinkles, as muscles adapt to regular face positions. Wear glasses or contacts to avoid squinting and smooth out your forehead instead of frowning when you're upset or annoyed.

## 152 WITCH HAZEL FACE FIRMER

Witch hazel can temporarily tighten the skin and give facial tissues a lift. Instead of using it neat, which can stress delicate skin, mix 1 teaspoon with 100g (3½ oz) of moisturizer and after two weeks you should see results.

## 153 RESIST DAMAGE WITH VITAMIN C

Antioxidant vitamin C in suncreens, moisturizers and capsules will help skin resist damage from sun, pollution and dryness so less wrinkles appear.

## 154 GO MARINE

Marine proteins, found in some creams and many supplements, can have skin-strengthening and -boosting properties, which may help reduce fine lines, wrinkles and sun-induced premature ageing.

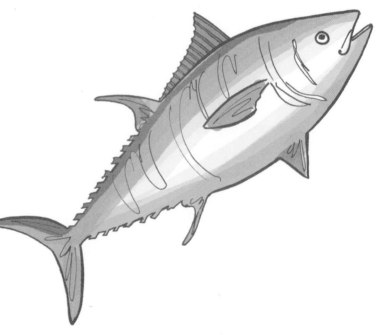

# 155 BE COOL IN SHADES

Sunglasses will stop lines developing around your eyes, caused by squinting against sun or harsh light. Problem areas are in cars and changes in light intensity between inside and outside. Wearing shades in winter, when the sun is lower, is important, too.

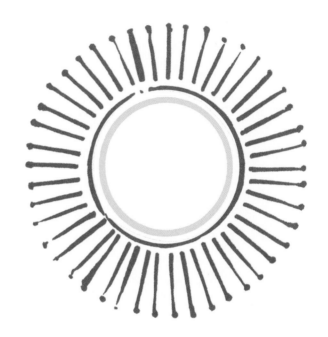

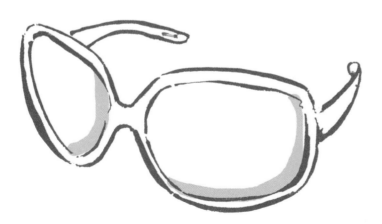

# base-ic rights

## 156 PAT IT OFF

After your make-up application, use a soft tissue to gently pat over your face. This will blend the make-up together and soften the look to help you appear natural without leaving you with uncovered patches.

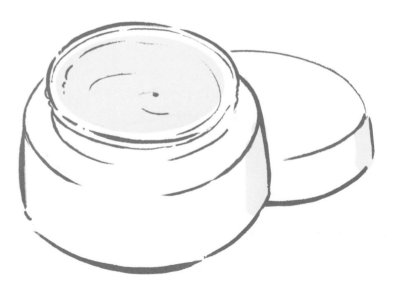

## 157 MAKE-UP WITH MINERALS

Because true mineral make-up contains no fillers, it furnishes long-lasting opaque coverage, while feeling weightless. This is a particular boon for individuals combating rosacea, as well as those who are healing after treatment.

## 158 DON'T CREASE UP

Applying eye creams and moisturizers before foundation lessens the probability of creasing because it smoothes out lines in the delicate under-eye area.

## 159 DITCH A DOUBLE CHIN

Get rid of your double chin by using a slightly darker shade of powder or foundation under your chin, which will make it appear to recede. Blend towards the back of the jawline to add definition.

## 160 DAMP IT UP

For even coverage apply foundation with a slightly damp sponge to spread the base around your face, or use a damp foundation brush for a more artistic approach.

## 161 TONE UP

Always choose a foundation that blends with your natural skin tone and never try to counteract your skin colour with a cosmetic. Asian skins have an underlying golden base so you need to choose yellow-based options. Ruddy complexions are best with ivory- or pink-based shades.

## 162 AVOID THE GREY FOR DARK SKINS

Too many foundations for dark and black skins are chalky and ashen. To find the right shade, look for rich colours in a sheer formulation that will allow your natural skin colour to shine through, while evening out pigmentation. Very matt formulas are the worst culprits for a greyish cast.

## 163 GO OIL-FREE

In warm, humid weather, skin is prone to producing more oil. Therefore the first port-of-call when summer comes round is an oil-free foundation. Oil-free liquid and sheer formulations are good matt, lightweight options that won't clog pores or leave shine.

## 164 BAKE THE CAKE

If your foundation is cakey or too dark, don't just add more and try to rub in. Instead, remove it with a tissue, working from the jaw and hairline outward with a sweeping motion.

## 165 CHOOSE A VERSATILE PRODUCT

Wet-dry foundations are adaptable for all skin types, especially oily and combination skins. They can be used in several ways – sponged on dry for a natural look, sponged on damp for coverage and for building up areas in thin layers, or used dry as a powder throughout the day.

## 166 TRY BEFORE YOU BUY

It's always a good idea to experiment with several different shades and brands before buying a new foundation.

## 167 GET A CUSTOM BLEND

To ensure you achieve the perfect shade of foundation, visit one of the beauty counters that will custom blend your very own shade for perfect results.

## 168 MAKEOVER YOUR MAKE-UP

If your skin darkens more than a shade or two during the summer, invest in a new foundation to match your skin tone. Blend them together for in-between colours, but stick to the same brand so the texture and formula remains the same.

## 169 GOODNIGHT, SWEET CREAMS

For maximum coverage, such as the kind of look you would choose for an evening party with low-level lighting, cream foundation is the best option.

## 170 MATT FOR MATURE

Matt foundation is a good for more mature skins, as it will cover imperfections and control shine without the skin looking too 'made-up' or overdone.

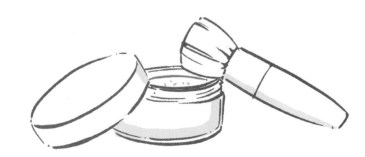

# 171 DON'T HIDE FROM THE LIGHT

Light-diffusing and -reflecting foundations deflect light away from fine lines and wrinkles, and contain micropigments that give a smooth finish. They have an instant anti-ageing effect and add a subtle glow.

# 172 MAKE FRIENDS WITH YOUR FRECKLES

Sheer foundation is best for freckled skin, which can look unnatural if none of the freckles are allowed to show through. Use a concealer first, then aim for the natural look – many people find freckles attractive.

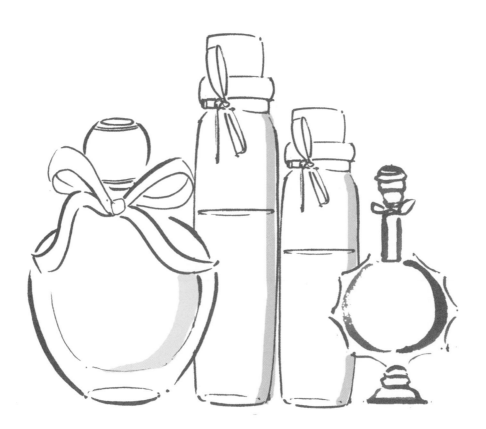

## 173 PREPARE YOUR CANVAS

Being heavy-handed with the moisturizer before you apply foundation can lead to streaking. Get the amounts right by applying a light application of moisturizer with a make-up sponge and leave it to dry for at least ten minutes before applying foundation and colour cosmetics.

## 174 LIKE LIQUID FOR DAY

For the sort of sheer-to-medium coverage that looks great in the daytime, try liquid foundations. These spread on easily and will last all day without becoming heavy or settling into fine lines. Always shake the bottle gently first to distribute the contents and apply to the centre of the face using light, dabbing movements with the finger-tips before gently blending outwards.

## 175 A WHITER SHADE OF PALE

If you prefer a pale, porcelain face with a flawless finish, use a white-coloured skin primer to give an all-over, even base before you apply a foundation. The primer will help avoid the need for touch-ups.

## 176 GET PUMP ACTION

If you can, choose a foundation in a tube or pump dispenser. These are good because the product can't slip back into the container after it has been exposed to air or touched, thus reducing the risk of contamination.

## 177 LONG FOR LONGLASTING?

A cream-to-powder foundation formula is a good option for dry and mature skins. It goes on as a rich, creamy moisturizer, but dries to a matt velvety finish that looks immaculate and provides good, longlasting coverage, which won't 'slip' or rub off during the day like many cream-based foundations.

## 178 USE AN INSTANT MIX

For a lighter look in seconds, mix your foundation with your daily moisturizer in the palm of your hand before applying it. This homemade, tinted moisturizer will give you a light, even coverage and is a perfect solution for summer months when you want a lighter weight of formula.

## 179 BRONZE AWAY REDS

If you have a ruddy complexion or uneven, browny-red skin tones, think about using a beige foundation or a bronzer to maintain the natural look while evening out skin tone. Many very pale foundations have a pinky undertone that will exacerbate redness.

## 180 NEUTRALIZE YELLOW

Get rid of yellow skin tones, especially in sallow skin around the eyes, using a violet skin correction colour.

## 181 GO GREEN TO REDUCE REDNESS

A green-coloured corrector under foundation can reduce cheek redness, but use sparingly and blend well, or you will make yourself look unnaturally pale.

## 182 BLEND, BLEND, BLEND

After you have applied your foundation, make sure you spend a few minutes blending it onto your jawline, hairline and slightly onto your neck. Spend twice as long on your foundation as you do on any other element of your make-up.

## 183 FACE FACTS ABOUT COMPACTS

Those with acne-prone skin should avoid compact foundations because the sponge can provide a breeding ground for bacteria and a heavy base may accentuate pimples and wrinkles. Go sheer instead.

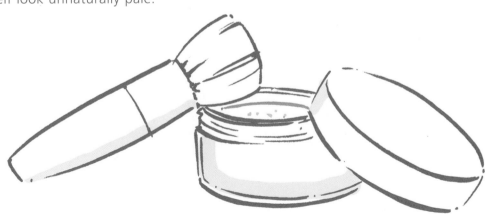

## 184 SPONGE IT OFF

Soak up excess foundation using a slightly damp, clean sponge. Press lightly onto the face, concentrating on the mouth, nose and hairline where it tends to collect.

## 185 PRIORITIZE AND MOISTURIZE

A layer of moisturizer provides a good base for make-up and protects the skin against clogging and dryness, caused by make-up soaking in. Not only will your make-up last longer, but your skin will feel fresher, too.

## 186 FORGET YOUR LINES

If you have lines on your forehead, apply a light, oil-based foundation and set with a little translucent, light reflective powder to hide the lines away.

## 187 BEWARE OF FACIAL HAIR

Try to avoid using thick foundations or powder on areas where you have facial hair. These products can cause the hairs to become more visible by forming a coating over them. If coverage is essential, wipe off any excess with a tissue.

## 188 CREAMY CHEEKS

If the skin on your cheeks is dry, go for a creamy or oil-based foundation that will help smooth out dry skin and stop make-up flaking and peeling. Moisturize first for best results.

## 189 YOUR DUTY TO BE DEWY

After you've applied foundation, to add a dewy glow, moisten a gauze pad or washcloth in a mild astringent like witch hazel and gently pat your face. The witch hazel will remove the matt look of your make-up and leave skin covered but radiant.

## 190 OPEN WIDE

When applying foundation, open your mouth to expose the neck area and allow you to blend your base over the jawline, to avoid an obvious line. Alternatively do it afterwards to check you've blended properly.

## 191 BE CLEVER WITH YOUR CLOTHES

Wearing light-coloured clothing helps to reflect light back onto the face, which can lighten dull skin and illuminate make-up.

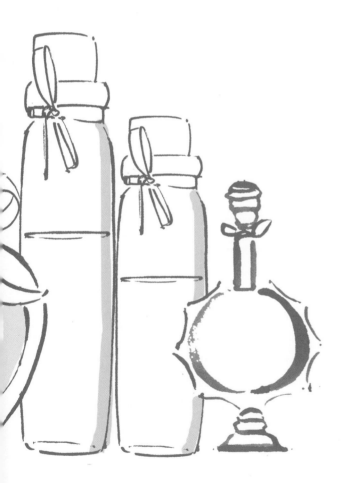

## 182 DON'T HOARD FOUNDATION

Throw foundation away if it starts to look or smell different, or if the ingredients start to separate. It may be out of date, which means it will have lost some of its texture and efficiency and will not glide on well.

## 183 LOOK FRESH AS A DAISY

Freshen foundation at the end of the day by dabbing moisturizer under the eyes and smoothing it across the cheekbones for a touch of added sheen.

## 184 TAKE CARE ON BROKEN SKIN

Be careful when using foundation near broken or infected skin as the infection could spread into the pot. Scoop a small amount onto a plastic dish, then put the container away so you don't accidentally contaminate the pot.

## 185 SPF IS ESSENTIAL

If you are not using a moisturizer with a SPF, make sure your foundation contains one – it is not necessary for both to have an SPF as you won't get increased protection.

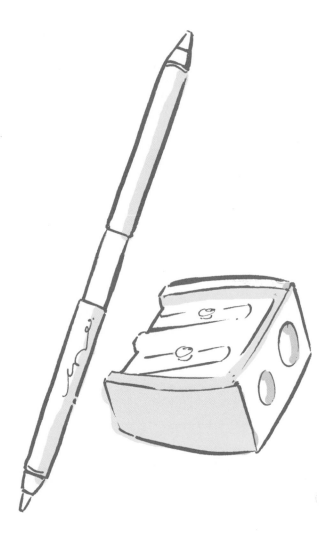

# brows

## 196 SHAPELY BROWS

To determine exactly where your brow should begin, imagine a vertical line or hold a make-up pencil straight alongside one nostril. Where the pencil lands by your brow is where it should begin. To work out where the brow should end, imagine a line from the outside of your nostril to the outer corner of your eye, extending out to your brow.

## 197 THREAD IT AWAY

Threading is a form of hair removal. It uses a small thread that is twisted around the eyebrow hairs to pull them out by the root. It is recommended for eyebrow shaping because it's less painful and not as harsh on the delicate skin than hot waxes.

## 198 DEFINE WITH A PENCIL

Pencils give the cleanest, most precise definition, but beware of drawing long lines. Instead, use light, feathery strokes to mimic hair growth.

## 199 GO TO A PROFESSIONAL

Take the easy route to perfect eyebrows by having your brows shaped by a beautician the first time you try re-shaping. All you then have to do is keep to the lines she's created for you, which takes much less time (and risk).

## 200 DIVIDE BY FOUR

For the best shape, think geometrically, as if the brow is divided into four sections along the length of the eye. The first three should head upward and the outer quarter should slant down.

## 201 BRUSH THOSE BROWS

An old toothbrush is excellent for brushing brows after pencilling in. Not only will it smooth down hairs, it will also soften pencil lines, leaving them looking more natural.

## 202 KEEP BROWS IN LINE

If you want your eyebrows to stay in place, add a coat of clear mascara or a little hairspray on the eyebrow groomer before brushing to the desired shape.

## 203 COMB IT UP

Comb brows upward before plucking or colouring in to make sure you preserve the natural browline. If your brows are very thick or long, trim the hairs that extend above the upper line of the arch.

## 204 POWDER IT RIGHT

Eyebrow powder should be one to two shades lighter than your hair colour. A matching colour to your hair can look overpowering on a face and anything much darker is just too severe.

## 205 KEEP IT SHARP

Sharpen your eyebrow pencil before every application to make sure you keep the high definition look you're after. You can always blend if lines are too sharp.

## 206 CATCH THE HIGHLIGHTS

To make brows appear higher and more defined, apply some highlighting powder or cream under the middle to outer edge of the eyebrow, which will add fullness to the eye area.

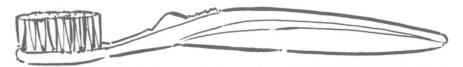

## 207 GO GREY GRACEFULLY

If you have grey, white, or salt and pepper hair, charcoal or slate grey are good shades to choose for brows, because they will look natural and still give definition.

## 208 KEEP TWEEZERS HANDY

Keep tweezers by the mirror for a daily tidy-up, plucking out just a few hairs as and when they appear. This will not only mean you stay looking tidy, but will stop overplucking and help you to keep your eyebrow shape.

## 209 JOIN THE BROWNIES

If you have red hair and eyebrows and want to colour them to give more emphasis to your face, beware of going too dark. Choose browns with deep red undertones instead, to blend with your hair.

## 210 BROWN IS THE NEW BLACK

For brunettes, apart from those with really dark hair, black can appear too harsh for eyebrows. Instead, choose a dark brown pencil, which will blend in more naturally.

## 211 CHOOSE LIGHT BROWN FOR BLONDE

If you have light hair and light skin, select light brown or taupe shades for eyebrows. These will contrast well with your skin without appearing too dark.

## 212 GET SHEEN WITH VASELINE

Tame wayward eyebrow hairs with a tiny amount of brow fixative or Vaseline after you've applied your brow colour. This will give them a bit of added shine as well as holding them in place.

## 213 POWDER AND PEAK

Powders give a soft effect and need minimal blending. To heighten the arch, apply an extra bit of colour at the highest peak to make it stand out.

## 214 PLUCK BEFORE BED

To avoid letting the whole world know you pluck your eyebrows, pluck last thing at night so the redness will have gone by the morning. After a bath or shower, when the skin is moist and the pores are open, is the best time to pluck.

## 215 KEEP 'EM HIGH

Never draw brows downward at the ends – this can have the effect of lowering your eyes and making them appear droopy. Instead, aim for a 'floating', winged effect to lift the face.

## 216 AVOID A CLOSE SHAVE

Never shave your eyebrows – it's hard to control and is likely to drag the skin, causing wrinkles. It also encourages hair to grow back blunt, which can bring attention to re-growth.

## 217 MAGNIFY TO BEAUTIFY

To get the best view of your brows, for even plucking, invest in a magnifying mirror and make sure the light falls evenly on both sides of your face to avoid uneven shapes caused by shadowing.

## 218 GET BELOW

Always pluck hairs from underneath the brow. Grasp hair as close to the root as possible and pull the hair out towards the temple in quick, firm strokes.

## 219 ENHANCE YOUR ARCHES

If you have a natural arch, work with it rather than creating a new one. If you need to create an arch, look into your eyes. The top arch of your eyebrow should fall directly above the outside of your iris for eye-opening results.

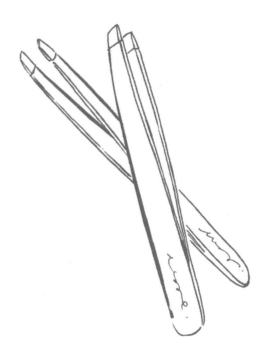

## 220 COLOURING IN

If you want to reshape your eyebrows, but are worried about making a mistake, fill in the area you want to preserve using an eyebrow pencil and pluck outside the edges. This way you won't over-pluck and you can perfect the shape first.

## 221 KEEP IT NATURAL

Never draw a browline above the natural one, it will look false and give you an unnaturally 'surprised' look. Instead, work with your natural lines and if necessary use a highlighter underneath to give brows a lift.

## 222 GET A PROFESSIONAL SHADE

If you want to permanently darken brows, visit a professional, who will be able to match up your shade perfectly for the most flattering results.

## 223 NOSE FIRST

When plucking and shaping eyebrows, start at the inner edge and around the bridge of the nose. Form a gentle, tapered round edge rather than a straight one.

## 224 TAKE THE TINT

Eyebrows should frame your face and eyes, but they may struggle to do this if they are too pale or have been bleached by the sun. Your brows may also go grey or lighter with age. Instead of filling in with powder, think of visiting a salon for professional brow tint which will usually last for four to six weeks.

## 225 STRETCH TO AVOID STING

Eyebrow tweezing can be painful. To avoid stinging and redness, stretch the skin gently upwards or between the fingers before plucking and pull out the hair quickly to avoid bruising. It is best to tweeze after a hot shower or bath and in the evening, to give your skin time to recover from any redness.

## 226 CIRCUMVENT YOUR CYCLE

Pain tolerance seems to be reduced just before and during the first few days of menstruation, so it's best to avoid these times if you're planning to re-shape eyebrows. Mid-cycle is the most pain-free time to pluck.

# cheeks

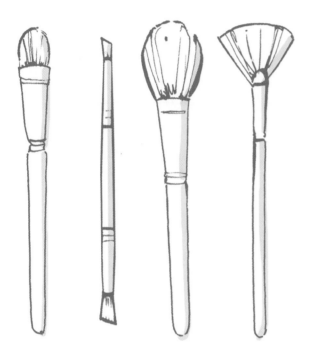

**228 KEEP TO THE CURVE**

Never apply blusher right up to the hairline, which is a sure fire way to make your face look unnaturally painted. Stop on the top curve of your cheekbone.

**229 BLOW AWAY BLUSHES**

To apply the perfect amount of blusher or bronzer to cheeks, load up the brush and then tap or blow off the excess. This will ensure you get ample coverage of colour without looking like a painted doll.

**230 BLUSH FOR TWO YEARS**

After two years, powders and powder blushers may start to develop a dry or 'slippery' texture. This is caused by too much mixing with natural oils from your skin. If this has happened to yours, it's time to invest in a new one.

**227 GIVE YOURSELF A SMILE**

To make blusher pay, smile into the mirror to find the apples of your cheeks, then brush the colour there in wide, sweeping movements for a natural, cheeky glow.

**231 DARKEN FOR DEFINITION**

To bring out your natural cheekbones, use a medium beige blush underneath to help the bones stand out – avoid dark colours or you will get a stripy look.

## 232 JOIN THE MAGIC CIRCLE

Soften the harshness of sharp cheekbones by applying blusher in circular motions on the apples of the cheeks. This will draw attention away from angled bones.

## 233 DISGUISE FULL CHEEKS

Use a light application of a slightly darker shade of powder than your foundation on the underside of cheekbones and blend out towards ears to sculpt some definition into round cheeks.

## 234 DON'T CLASH LIPS AND CHEEKS

Choose a cheek colour that blends with the colour on your lips or your natural lip colour to avoid clashing and looking 'overdone'. Or stick to skin tones if you're going bright.

## 235 BLOT AND BRONZE

Before applying bronzer, blot your skin with blotting papers or a clean tissue. This will give the skin an even surface and ensure that the bronzer doesn't end up in blotches.

## 236 LEAVE THE CREAM TO THE CAT

If your skin is oily, steer clear of cream blushers, which can give cheeks a shiny look and make skin elsewhere on the face appear oilier as a result.

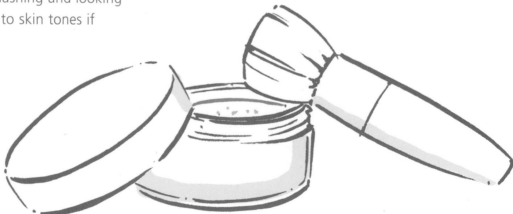

## 237 DON'T FREAK OVER STREAKS

If your blusher looks streaky or stripy, or if you have over coloured, don't be tempted to add more colour to even out the stripe. The only way to deal with it is to remove some colour with a tissue and dust a little translucent powder over cheeks.

## 238 USE GEL TO LOOK WELL

For a natural cheek colour, particularly over sheer tinted moisturizers, use cheek gel instead of powder blusher. Gel gives a healthy, translucent flush to the skin.

## 239 GLOW WITHOUT GOING OVERBOARD

When you want to add warmth to the skin, particularly in the daytime, use a light to medium bronzing powder instead of your standard blush.

## 240 BE A PEACH BABE

Choose soft natural pinks, beiges and tawny peaches for daytime. These will blend with the tones in natural daylight and avoid making you look overdone. Go brighter and cooler at night for definition.

## 241 LEAVE IT TILL LAST

For super-smooth results with no streaking, particularly for evening looks, apply blusher after powder. This will form a smooth, natural base that the colour can cling to.

## 242 CREATE CHEEKBONES

Cheekbones are best defined with highlighter rather than blusher, which can cause overcolouring. Blend a line of highlighter along the top edges of your cheekbones and a line of shade underneath to help them stand to attention.

## 243 GET IT RIGHT ON YOUR WRIST

Look for the most natural blush colour you can find. Try it on the inside of your wrist when choosing – if it looks natural here, it will look natural on your cheeks.

## 244 THE FUTURE IS NOT ORANGE

When choosing a bronzer, make sure it doesn't appear too orange or frosted. A little shimmer goes a long way; too much can make skin look unnatural and harsh, especially on mature skin.

## 245 TWO WILL DO

Never go more than two shades darker than your natural skin tone. Bronzers are meant to warm your skin as if you have a natural glow, rather than adding colour.

## 246 GO EASY ON BASE

Too much foundation can leave your bronzer looking 'muddy' and artificial, ruining the natural glow effect you are aiming for. If you feel you really need foundation, try a tinted moisturizer or sheer base instead.

## 247 HOW TO DO DEWY

Powder bronzers are best for oily complexions. If your skin is dry or you like a dewy finish, choose a cream, stick or gel to achieve your colour.

## 248 BLUSH IT UP

For lighter complexions, use a small amount of bronze on your cheeks and forehead. Follow this with a touch of pink or rose blush on the apples of your cheeks, for a natural-looking flush.

## 249 FINGER PAINTING

Cream, stick and liquid bronzers should be applied using your fingers. Dab them onto the apples of your cheeks and blend, using circular motions, toward the hairline. Leftover colour can be very lightly dabbed onto the bridge of the nose, on the temples and even on the collarbone.

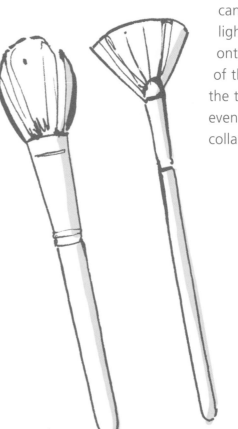

### 250 COLOUR ON THE GO

If you're in a rush and need a quick touch up, invest in an all-in-one lip/eye/blush in a crayon, stick or gel to give you a colour lift anytime and anywhere.

# conceal it

### 251 DON'T GO TOO LIGHT

The most common mistake women make when applying concealer is choosing a colour that is too light. This merely achieves the opposite effect by actually highlighting the problem, especially if you're using it to cover under-eye circles.

### 252 CONCEAL DARK CIRCLES

Concealer is the most important step in banishing dark circles and preparing the skin for a perfectly even base. Gently pat a light reflecting creamy concealer above and below the eye area to disguise imperfections. Avoid powdery sticks that can pull the skin.

### 253 CORRECT RIDGES WITH CONCEALER

If you don't like the hollow of your chin or think your nose ridges are too prominent, correct them using a few dabs of concealer just as you would with a spot or blemish. Finish with a little translucent powder.

### 254 STICK IT TO LAST

Stick concealer lasts the longest of any type because it's less prone to drying out or discolouring over time. Liquid-based concealers may start to separate or go lumpy when they're past their date.

### 255 COVER IT UP WITH GOLD

For concealing under-eye circles, which can often appear bluish in colour, choose a gold-based, warm-toned concealer that will counteract the blue and help you hide them.

### 256 COVER YOUR EYES

If you're covering up under-eye circles, don't just put the concealer under the eye, which can give you a 'striped' look. Instead, cover the whole eye area and set with a light dusting of powder.

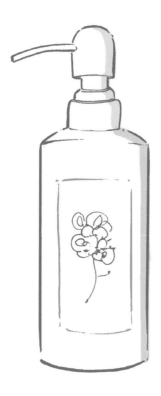

**257** **HIDE YOUR NOSE**

To slim down a wide nose, use highlighter and blend a soft line down the centre of the nose, then add a contour shade (a darker powder or non-shimmery bronzer) to the outside of the nose and blend together well.

**258** **CONCEAL ALL DAY**

Apply foundation before camouflaging problem areas with a cream concealer. Finally, dot with translucent powder to hold the concealer in place all day long.

**259** **CONCEAL WITH A COTTON BUD**

Using a cotton bud or small, pointed concealer brush, apply a dot of thick concealer to the centre of the blemish, then lightly spread it to cover. Brush over with translucent powder.

**260** **COVER UP PIMPLES**

It's fine to wear make-up if you have pimples, provided that it is not an allergic reaction to that particular brand. The important thing is to remember to cleanse well at the end of the day.

**261** **CONCEAL AFTER FOUNDATION**

Apply foundation first and then your concealer. Foundation will hide three quarters of all the discolourations you see on a bare face. Finish with concealers on the most obvious areas.

### 262 BANISH SPOTS WITH BASE

Give spots, patches of discolouration and blemishes their own covering of foundation and allow to dry before applying the same base all over your face. Use the thicker foundation that has settled around the bottleneck and lid of your bottle, as it is similar in consistency to a concealer.

# eye care

### 263 HORSE AROUND

For reducing under-eye bags, creams containing vitamin K and horse chestnut are thought to exert beneficial effects by reducing puffiness and blood flow under the thin skin of the area.

### 264 GO GENTLY INTO THE NIGHT

When you apply night cream under your eyes, do so gently. Use your fourth finger (which is the weakest) and pat the cream back and forth under the eye, starting at the outer corner and working inward.

### 265 KEEP IT LOW

Don't put eye cream on your upper lids before bedtime or you'll wake up with puffy lids. The cream will prevent the delicate skin in the area from breathing.

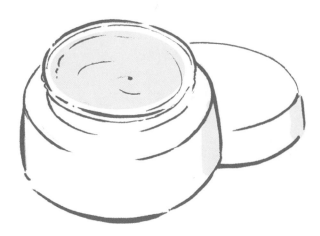

### 266 SOOTHE EYES WITH CUCUMBER

Place a slice of cucumber on each eyelid for 10–15 minutes to allow the high water and mineral content of the cucumber to be absorbed into your delicate eye skin.

### 267 USE AN EXTRA PILLOW

Using an extra pillow can help avoid puffy morning eyes by assisting fluid to drain out of the face by angling it downward. If your neck gets sore, move the pillow under your chest or shoulders.

### 268 WAKE UP EYES WITH AYURVEDA

To keep your peepers perky with an Ayurvedic remedy, sprinkle cold water ten times over tired eyes (keeping them open) morning and night. If you wear contact lenses, do this before you put them in!

# eyeliner

### 269 KEEP SPARKLE SUBTLE

For subtle sparkle, choose a glitter eyeliner with some added glitter that will give you a little bit of extra glamour. Don't be tempted to use other sparkly products on your eyes at the same time though.

### 270 FLATTEN OUT ROUND EYES

Make like a cat by flattening round eyes. Apply a liner only to the top lashes from the inner to the outer corners of the eye to give it a more elongated appearance.

### 271 DON'T BE BLUNT

Sharpen your eye pencil every time you use it. This prevents eye bacteria building up on the round, blunt end, which could spread to other parts of your eyes. It will also help you achieve high definition as blunt ends are much harder to control.

## 272 HOT SMOKE

Create a smokey evening look by running your eye pencil under hot water before you apply it for a deeper, smudgy look.

## 273 SMOKE IT OUT

For a natural smokey look, whatever colour your eyeliner pencil is, smudge it in tiny circular motions that will provide you with a naturally blended line.

## 274 BE A KOHL KITTEN

Create that classic sex kitten effect on the eyes by lining the top and bottom lash lines to the outer corners in a classic black kohl pencil. Set this off with a few lashings of curl-enhancing mascara.

## 275 MODERNIZE YOUR EYES

Instead of using eyeliner for daily make-up, use powder eyeshadow applied with a very narrow brush to give a smokey, modern appearance to the edge of eyes. Smudge further if necessary with a larger brush. Alternatively, use the powder wet for a sharper line of colour.

## 276 IT'S COOL TO BE SHARP

Eyeliners will sharpen better after a few hours in the fridge – the cold makes the ends firmer and less prone to stickiness. Let them warm up to room temperature before you use them or they'll be too hard.

## 277 STAY OUTSIDE

Unless you're blessed with almond-shaped eyes, stick to using eyeliner on the outside rather than inside the lash line. Applying it inside will make your peepers seem smaller and dull their colour.

## 278 HIDE EYE CIRCLES

To draw attention away from under-eye bags or circles, avoid applying eyeliner or mascara to lower lashes, which could draw attention downward instead of up.

## 279 WIDEN WITH WHITE

To give your eyes the appearance of being wider set, line the inside of the bottom rim of your eyes with a soft white eyeliner pencil. This will also give you a fresher, younger look.

## 280 GO FOR THE TILT

To apply liner to your upper lash line, tip your head back and look down into a mirror. Rest a slightly blunted pencil tip on the lash line and push between your lashes, from inside to outside.

## 281 COOL FOR KOHL

Kohl pencils are ideal for summer days because they give a slightly waxy, soft look, which is simple and natural. For a clean look, use thin kohl pencils rather than crayons, which can be messier.

## 282 BE ALL WHITE

White liner can be a real beauty secret for widening eyes and looking younger. Etch it along the inner rim to brighten eyes and reduce redness. Choose a white that's flecked with gold or rose tones.

## 283 FEATHER IT WELL

Avoid sharp, hard lines around your eyes, which looks dated and obvious, by feathering eyeliner and blending it with a little powder for a smokey look.

## 284 KEEP LIQUID THIN

Liquid eyeliners are great for a defined evening look, but don't extend the line beyond the natural corner of the eye and keep it thin for the most glamorous look. If you have trouble keeping steady, try making three dashes – at the inner, middle and outer corners, then joining them up.

# eyeshadow

## 285 COMPLEMENT, DON'T COLOUR

The purpose of eyeshadow is to shape and accentuate the eye, not colour it. Even if you're going bright, choose tones that accentuate your natural shades.

## 286 DAYLIGHT IS BRIGHT ENOUGH

Steer clear of bright eyeshadow or coloured mascara in the daytime because harsh sunlight can make the colours appear even brighter, washing out your face and eyes. Leave the bright colours for creating a dazzling looks in the evening.

## 287 GET BRAND SAVVY

If you're using two shades of powdered eyeshadow, use the same brand, as they are more likely to be of the same formula, thus easier to blend with each other.

## 288 LINE UP THE BROWN

For paler skins, light browns and taupe eyeliners work best because they enhance the natural tones of the eye without overpowering the surrounding skin.

## 289 SPARKLE IT UP WITH GOLD AND BRONZE

For evenings, there are several illuminating, loose and pressed powders on the market, which add a bit of sparkle with both gold and bronze flecked effects.

## 290 BE A ONE-TRICK WONDER

As a general rule, let your eyes or your lips do the talking – not both. This doesn't mean neglecting either area, just plump for a more natural look for one and use stronger make-up on the other. Usually you will want to concentrate on your best feature.

## 291 KEEP IT NEUTRAL

Do use flattering neutrals to contour and highlight your eyes for a timeless daytime look that will last. For eyeliners, stick to classic colours like black, navy or brown.

## 292 LOOK LIVELY

For sparkling whites of eyes, go for cooler shades near the corner of the eyes, where the colour is nearest the eyeball. Avoid yellows and reds in this area, which can make your eyes look sickly.

## 293 GREEN UP THE BLUE

If you have blue eyes, enhance their natural colour with a subtle green eyeshadow rather than blue – it will bring out the blue eye colour without being overpowering.

## 294 PROHIBIT POWDER ON PARCHED SKIN

If your skin is dry, aged or wrinkled, avoid powder eyeshadows and base products, which can accentuate wrinkles. Opt for lightweight creams instead, which will keep skin looking smooth and even.

## 295 TOUCH IT UP

If you're in a hurry, add extra touches of cream or gel-type eyeshadow with the tip of your middle finger. Just a dot of the product, applied lightly, should work just fine.

## 296 GLOW FOR GOLD

Give eyes a gorgeous glistening glow for summer by dusting a shimmer golden bronzer or loose gold dust over eyelids and cheekbones. To add intensity, highlight the outer corners of your eyes with a darker copper or brown eyeshadow.

## 297 CREAMS INCREASE CREASES

Lightly powder lids before eyeshadow to keep them crease-proof longer. If you're prone to creasing, avoid cream colours in favour of silky powders.

## 298 SOFTEN UP FROGGY EYES

If you have large, prominent eyes, do not use loud or bright colours, which will over-emphasize their fullness. Go for soft shades and neutrals instead.

## 299 FOIL SPILLS

Apply a dusting of loose powder directly under-eye area before you apply your eyeshadow. Afterwards, whisk away the powder from under your eyes with a brush and it will take eyeshadow fallout with it.

## 300 DON'T OVERDO THE SHIMMER

Be careful with shimmery products, especially on your eyelids, as they tend to collect in the creases. They are best left for evening, where they won't have to hold the look for as long.

## 301 BRING EYES OUT WITH LIGHT

On deep-set eyes, choose shadow colours that are on the light side of the colour spectrum, particularly on the bit of lid directly above the eye, which will make them appear more prominent.

## 302 SWEEP IT UP

After you've applied foundation sweep a darker shade of bronzer or powder from the outside top edge of your eyebrow toward your hairline. This will give your eyes the illusion of being higher and wider.

### 303 LIGHTEN YOUR INNER CORNERS

Often the inner corner of your eye, near the nose, is the darkest part and can drag down your whole face. If you use a slightly lighter shadow or eye pencil on this area, it will bring it out of the dark and help your eyes look bigger, too.

### 304 GO GOLD FOR HIGHLIGHTS

For a glamorous evening look use silver and gold eyeshadows as highlights for the browbone. Stick to the area under the brow and don't take the highlighter out too far towards your temple, which can appear too obvious.

### 305 LONG MAY IT LAST

If you want your eyeshadow to last all day, prime your eyelids with a thin layer of foundation before applying your eye colour. If you forgo shadow for a bare look, it will also help your eyelids blend in with the skin tone on the rest of your face, in which case using mascara will be necessary to give your eyes some definition.

# face masks

### 306 EGGS-ELEVEN

Eggs make masks to suit all skin types. An egg white whipped and patted on the skin will tighten and tone. The whole egg, beaten, has softening properties as well. Add egg to any mask for an 'eggstra' treat!

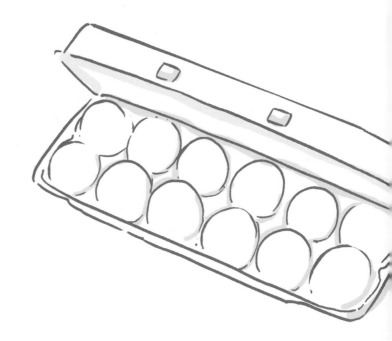

### 307 MASKS ARE ANTI-AGEING

For mature skin, masks can deliver a burst of temporary anti-ageing ingredients that instantly softens and smoothes lines. Often the firming effects can last for several days.

### 308 GO EASY FOR SENSITIVE SKIN

If you find your skin reacts badly to masks, but you still want to use them, try those with gentler ingredients like camomile and cucumber, and avoid lanolin, which can often cause reactions.

### 309 BE A SMOOTH-SKINNED HONEY

Honey and almond flour, mixed together into a paste, is an excellent scrub for oily skin because of honey's antiseptic properties and the high levels of vitamins they both contain. Its graininess makes it an excellent gentle exfoliator.

## 310 POST-MASK MOISTURE BOOST

Always moisturize directly after using a mask, unless the mask is a leave-on product and you are instructed to rub in the residue. With dead skin cells sloughed off and pores unclogged, your moisturizer will sink in more deeply and have greater penetrating results.

## 311 CLEANSE BEFORE YOU COVER

You wouldn't polish a dirty floor and neither should you put a mask on a dirty face. You'll only get the full benefits if you apply the mask to cleansed skin, which will allow your face to absorb more of the ingredients in the mask.

## 312 FINISH WELL

If you didn't exfoliate before a mask, finish by removing the mask using a warm, wet face cloth in gentle circular movements. This will act as a gentle exfoliant and leave skin instantly brighter and clearer-looking. However do not use a scrub or product exfoliator at this stage as you do not want to strip the skin.

## 313 BOSH BLACKHEADS

For a homemade way to banish blackheads, combine equal amounts of baking soda and water in your hands to form a paste, then rub the mixture gently into skin, on the affected areas only, for two to three minutes. Finally rinse off.

## 314 WATERMELON CLEANSING

Make yourself a cleansing and clarifying face mask using watermelon, which clears the skin of blemishes and leaves it feeling fresh and clear. Apply the pure juice to your face, leave it on for 15 minutes and then splash with cold water to remove it.

## 315 MUD, GLORIOUS MUD

Oily skin responds well to clay- or mud-based masks, but never use them on dry skin as they are too harsh. When the mask is removed, surface dirt, oil and dead skin cells adhere to the clay and are rinsed away with the mask. If you suffer from an oily T-zone but dry cheeks, apply the mud mask only in the T-zone area and use a gentle moisturizing mask for the cheeks.

### 316 BREW UP A STORM

For oily skin, a brewer's yeast mask can help tone without drying out. Mix a teaspoon of brewer's yeast with enough natural yogurt to make a loose, thin mixture. Pat this thoroughly into the oily areas and allow it to dry on the skin. After 15–20 minutes, rinse off with warm water, then cool and blot dry.

### 317 BANANAS FOR SMOOTH SKIN

Banana is one of the best ingredients for an anti-wrinkle treatment because of its vitamins, minerals and smooth, soothing consistency. Mash down two or three slices with a little milk. Apply all over your face and leave for 15–20 minutes before rinsing off with warm water.

### 318 GO GENTLY WITH CUCUMBER

For gentle rehydration for sensitive skins, combine half a cucumber, scooped out of its skin, one tablespoon of yogurt, a few strawberries, and one teaspoon of honey. Apply to your face and allow to dry, then gently wipe off.

### 319 HIT BLEMISHES WITH A CARROT STICK

A carrot mask can work wonders for blemished complexions. Use a small, raw carrot mashed to a smooth paste or boil one in a little water and mash it. Then pat the mask all over the blemished areas and leave on for 15–20 minutes. Rinse and pat dry.

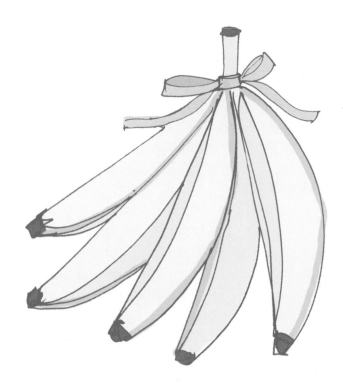

## 320 MIX UP A VITAMIN BLEND

Create a replenishing face mask with the flesh of one avocado, a little orange juice, honey, molasses and a few drops of camomile essential oil whizzed together in a blender to give your skin a vitamin boost.

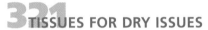

## 321 TISSUES FOR DRY ISSUES

Masks for dry skin can be tissued off if your skin is extra-dry, so a thin film of the moisture stays behind quenching skin for hours afterwards. Be careful not to leave too much product on as it can clog pores.

## 322 DO A PATCH TEST

People with sensitive skin should take care when using masks. Test a small amount of the mask on the area behind your ear and watch for 24 hours to see if there's a reaction. Always remove masks immediately if you feel tingling or burning.

## 323 LAY IT ON THICK

Masks work best when coverage is generous, so don't be afraid to use a thicker application. This is one case when trying to skimp is a false economy because the mask won't do as much for the skin if it's thin and you'll only be more tempted to use it more often.

## 324 PACK IT WITH PETALS

Prepare a rose face mask by grinding a handful of petals into a paste with a little milk and, if desired, a teaspoon of honey. Apply to clean skin and leave for 15–25 minutes. Wash the paste off with plain water (no soap) and your complexion will be smooth, soft and glowing.

## 325 GIVE YOURSELF A GRAPE BOOST

Forget expensive lotions – grape juice makes an excellent cleanser for any skin type. Simply split one or two large grapes, remove their pips and rub the flesh over your face and neck for an instant, antioxidant cleanser. Rinse off with cool water.

# highlighters

### 326 DON'T SWEAT IT

Illuminators and highlighters are great for picking out areas you want to highlight, but take care when applying them as a skin base or you could end up looking as if you have a sweaty face. Mix a tiny amount with your usual foundation for best results.

### 327 DOTS OF LIGHT

Dots of highlighter have a powerful illuminating effect. Apply a dot of high-lighter in the inner corners of the eyes, on the lips or on the tip of the nose to add shine and definition to your face.

### 328 BE A RADIANT WOMAN

A perfect remedy for hungover skin, radiance boosters are applied after moisturizer and before foundation, but they also work well when patted over make-up for a quick, mid-day perk-up. They add instant glow, making you appear more wide-awake and fresher.

### 329 BOOST WITH A SPRITZ

Spritzing rosewater or a water spray over make-up is an instant reviver. It rehydrates skin and adds a natural glow, helping to get that natural dewy look without adding any extra product.

### 330 GOLDEN GIRLS

Gold-based highlighters are great in the summer when applied on top of bare skin or for darker complexions. In the cooler winter light, however, choose the pink versions that will give the same effect.

### 331 SHIMMER IT UP

Mixing a few drops of highlighter or shimmer lotion into liquid foundation gives a subtle gleam, which you can use to highlight areas such as cheekbones, eyebrows and the upper lip.

### 332 CHOOSE YOUR PRODUCT

Many highlighters and illuminators come as creams, balms, multipurpose sticks and tubes for applying in specific areas or blending in all over the face.

## 333 DON'T SHIMMER WITH DISCO GLITTER

For a versatile choice, choose a fine, loose powder shimmer that you can apply with a blusher brush, not only on the face but also on the shoulders, décolletage and legs. These are fine, high-grade particles and a million miles away from those glittery disco powders for teens.

## 334 LOOK WHERE THE LIGHT HITS

Apply highlighter on those areas that are directly hit by daylight, such as the tops of the cheekbones and the temples. Stand in front of a mirror in a bright light to test the best areas.

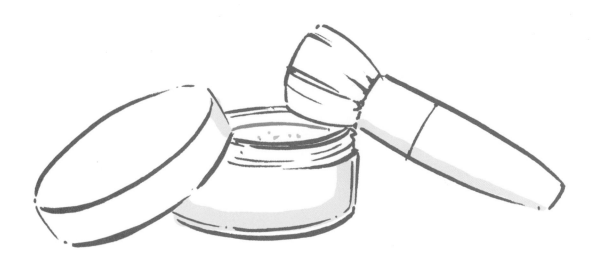

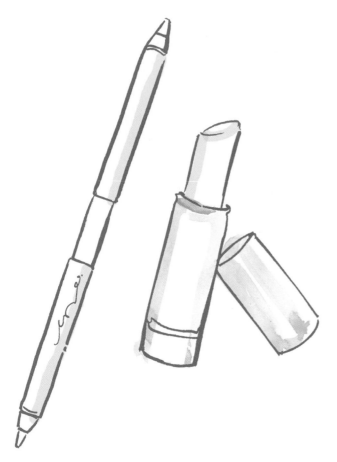

# lips

### 335 PLUMP UP YOUR LIPS

Newly developed lip plumping glosses, with swelling ingredients like cinnamon and menthol, claim to temporarily inflate the pout, mimicking the effects of permanent surgical lip fillers like collagen and hyalauronic acid.

### 336 PEAK A POUT

Instead of completely outlining the lips, for a bigger pout just pencil in the cupid's bow, the centre of the bottom lip, and the corners of the mouth with a natural shade. This will enhance the shape of your lips, bringing attention to the edges and giving them a fuller appearance.

### 337 KEEP LIPSTICK OFF YOUR TEETH!

Once you've applied your lipstick, put your forefinger in your mouth and then (just like a lollipop) slowly pull it out. All the lipstick that would have ended up on your teeth will have been successfully removed and you will be able to smile with security.

## 338 AFRAID OF THE DARK

Don't use a lipliner much darker than your lipstick to define your lips.

## 339 BRUSH UP YOUR LIP SKILLS

For the ultimate in flawless lipstick application, use a specially designed lip brush – it's the best way to avoid finishing up with too much lipstick. Simply blot with a single ply of tissue after each application and build-up the colour until you get the result you're looking for.

## 340 DON'T LICK YOUR LIPS

Don't be tempted to lick dry, cracked or chapped lips, which can be caused by harsh conditions or dehydration, as this will only make them dryer. Take a drink of water and use a lip balm or moisturizer to restore plumpness instead.

## 341 ADDRESS YOUR DRYNESS

Very matt and longwearing lipsticks can be quite dry and lacking in oil. If your lips are prone to dryness, creamy formulas are a lot more flattering.

## 342 DO 3D LIPS

Use your light brown eye pencil to line lips. Apply a bit more on the inside corners of the lip and on both top and bottom to create depth on the outside of the lips and a 3D effect lip.

## 343 GLOSS AND BE GONE

Lip gloss isn't as longlasting as lipstick because it is formulated in a different way and is prone to drying. If it changes scent, texture, or looks or feels different on your lips, it's time for a change.

## 344 MAKE DO AND BLEND

If you can't find the right shade, mix it up by using your existing lipsticks to create new colours. Simply blend the colours onto the back of your hand with a lip brush and apply directly to your lips.

## 345 POUT IT UP

Create a pretty pout by first applying your lip colour with a lip brush, then using a lip pencil afterwards in a complementary colour. Be sure to follow the natural line of your lips.

### 346 GET LUSCIOUS LIPS

Just as your face needs regular moisturizing, so too do your lips. Before you go to bed is the perfect time to really allow the moisture to sink in. Before you go to sleep, apply a large dose of your favourite lip balm and wake up in the morning with a perfectly rehydrated pout.

### 347 FIGHT FEATHERING

To prevent lipstick from feathering, line your mouth with a lip pencil, which will fill in lines and help to keep colour intact.

### 348 MAKE SURE YOU MATCH

Always choose a lipliner that matches your lip colour, then if your lipstick wears off you won't look overdone.

### 349 BE A GOOD CHAP

Use a Chapstick as a lip primer under colour. The waxiness smoothes the lip surface, fills tiny lines and will help hold the colour for longer. This is particularly useful under matt colours, which can add to the appearance of dryness.

### 350 LIP IT UP

If you're wearing make-up, always apply something to your lips, even if it's just a bit of lipliner and gloss, to make sure you look finished.

### 351 TOUCH BASE WITH YOUR LIPSTICK

To form a perfect lipstick base, apply a light covering of foundation with a wet sponge and allow to dry. This will even out underlying skin tone and allow lipstick to stay on for longer.

### 352 FINGERTIP TESTER

When choosing a lipstick, never apply the tester directly to your lips. For hygiene reasons the best place to test is your fingertips, where the colour and texture of skin is closest to your lips.

### 353 EVEN IT OUT

Even out uneven upper and lower lips by using lipliner only on the thinner one to create the appearance of equality. Alternatively opt for a slightly darker shade on the thinner one to boost visibility.

## 354 THINK OF YOUR SKIN

Don't be tempted to match lipstick to clothes instead of skin colour – go for shades that flatter your complexion rather than those that match your outfit for the most flattering results.

## 355 STEM BLEEDING WITH POWDER

To avoid your lip colour bleeding, after applying lipstick, dot powder at the upper and lower corners of the mouth, at the outside edge, to fill in lines. Brush away excess powder.

## 356 BE A GLOSS LEADER

Create fullness with a spot of gloss in the middle of the mouth, particularly on the upper lips, which will appear fuller as a result.

## 357 DON'T BE SHY OF BIG LIPS

If your lips are large, don't be shy; promote them as a star feature using a deep coloured, matt lipstick. Avoid gloss and really bright colours, which can overly increase the voluptuous effect.

## 358 SAY IT BRIGHT

Lightweight brightening creams can give thin lips a natural-looking pout if blended over the lip line before using lipstick or gloss.

## 359 GOLDEN DELICIOUS

For an instant, glammed-up evening look apply a small amount of gold-coloured or sparkly gloss over your daytime lipstick to get you in the mood.

## 360 NICE AND EVEN

Some women naturally have uneven amounts of colour in their lips. To neutralize natural lip colour, dot foundation on your lips and blot before applying colour.

## 361 GO THE EXTRA SMILE

Make your lips look fuller by using a pale or frosty lipstick and finish with a splash of gloss in the middle of your mouth to achieve the perfect pout.

## 362 SEAL IT WITH AN E

To seal in lipstick instantly, prick a vitamin E capsule and slick it over your lip colour.

## 363 STRIVE FOR EQUALITY

If you have a thinner top lip, you can help it stand out more by applying a slick of gloss to the top lip only to accentuate it, then blotting gently onto the lower lip.

## 364 GET FLAWLESS COLOUR

To achieve the exact colour of the lipstick on your lips, apply a nude lip pencil to your lips before the lipstick. It will also help keep the lipstick in place for longer and reduce the chances of smudging.

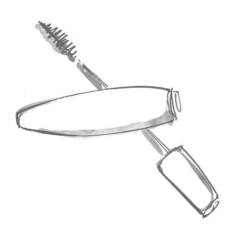

# mascara

## 365 WEAR LIGHT LAYERS

Three or four coats of thinly applied mascara are more alluring and natural-looking than one or two clumpy applications. When it comes to eyelashes, the thinner the better!

## 366 GO WIDE

Concentrate mascara application on the outside of the eye – this will help to widen eyes and bring attention to the curved edges, making them appear more alluring.

## 367 KEEP IT UP TOP

Always use less mascara on your lower lashes, this will naturally 'lift' your eyes. Too much on lower lashes can make eyes look droopy.

## 368 MIRROR YOUR MASCARA

To apply mascara easily, look down into a mirror and brush through lashes from roots to tips, first on top then on the underneath of lashes. This will help avoid the brush hitting the eyelid.

### 369 ONE COAT AT A TIME

Apply one coat of mascara carefully and wait for it to dry before considering a second one. You may only need one application, this way, you'll avoid clogging.

### 370 LUBRICATE YOUR LASHES

Rub Vaseline, baby oil or eyelash conditioner into eyelashes overnight (do this with your eyes closed). This will will help keep your lashes conditioned and prevent any breakage of the ends.

### 371 CULL OLD MASCARA

If you've had your mascara for more than three or four months, it's time to throw it out and get a new one. Over this time, the colour will dry out and prevent you being able to put on smooth, even coats.

### 372 WARM UP MASCARA

If your mascara thickens when it reaches the end of the tube, place the sealed tube in warm water for a few minutes to help make the mascara thinner.

### 373 SPURN THE CHURN

Don't churn your mascara wand around in the mascara vial, it could introduce air and make it clog. A simple in-and-out movement will do, and keep the top on whenever it's not in use.

### 374 BE STILL

Don't be tempted to apply mascara or liner if you're on the move, in a car or on a train, however late you are. It's impossible to make an even job of it, however steady your hand.

### 375 TRIM YOUR FALSIES

Trim false eyelashes before you apply them to mimic the natural shape of your eyelashes and to define your eyes. Make the outer edges longer for eye-widening results.

## 376 GET BEDROOM EYES

False lashes have improved dramatically and salons now offer extensions that can last up to three months. They are glued on lash by lash and offer fantastic length and colour, but you must follow strict care guidelines.

## 377 BRUSH AWAY CLOGS

If you don't have a mascara comb to hand, get rid of nasty looking clogs by following your mascara application with a quick brush through with an old, washed-and-dried mascara wand.

## 378 DON'T ADD WATER

Never add water or other liquid to mascara to keep it from drying out, as this can cause the preservative to become diluted and therefore offer less protection against germs and bacteria.

## 379 GET THE WIGGLES

When applying mascara, wiggle your wand on the base of the lashes. It's the mascara near the roots – not the tips – that gives the illusion of length and thickness.

## 380 MONOGAMOUS MASCARA

Never share mascara – this is the most common way to pass on eye infections such as conjunctivitis. Also don't use the same mascara if you've just had an eye infection, which could re-introduce the infection or affect the other eye.

## 381 WASH BEFORE THE WAND

Always wash your hands before applying mascara to cut down the risk of passing on bacteria with your hands, especially if you're one of those people who uses their hands to touch their eye area while they apply.

## 382 STROKE IT ON

For the smoothest results, stroke on colour in smooth strokes, from root to tip and in an upward motion. Avoid side-to-side movements, which can apply it too thickly.

## 383 PLUM IT UP

For a different look on dark lashes, go for a top coat of plum mascara to bring out the colour of dark hair and eyes. Applying it over black is an excellent evening option.

### 384 PREVENT OVERLOAD

When you first buy mascara it's thinner and more liquid, which means it goes on heavier. To avoid over-doing it, and to ensure a lighter covering, allow the wand to dry for a few seconds in the air before you apply.

### 385 WORK THE WAND

First, apply mascara to the middle and inner lashes using upward strokes, then concentrate on the outer lashes, sweeping out at a 45-degree angle to enhance the outer edge of the eye.

### 386 GO TOP AND BOTTOM

Apply mascara to the tops of the lashes as well as the underneath to give them a thicker, more defined look. This is especially good for evening looks.

### 387 CURL BEFORE YOU COAT

Curl your lashes before you apply mascara, then the roots will be easier to get at and you can ensure a more effective, all-over covering of colour.

### 388 KINKS AND CURLS

Nothing opens up eyes more than curling the eyelashes. Curl at the base first, then at the halfway point to finish. Hold for about ten seconds, and always curl on clean lashes. Heat a metal curler under a hot hairdryer for a few seconds first to replicate the effects of a heated eyelash curler.

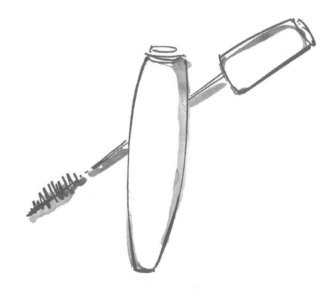

### 389 GET RIDGES

Choosing a mascara applicator with ridges rather than bristles can help avoid clogs by ensuring an even coating. Mascara can get stuck in bristles, which are then passed on to your lashes.

### 390 BLACK IS FOR DARK LADIES

As a rule, the only people who look really good in black mascara are those with deep brunette hair and darker skins, which can take the harsh contrast of black.

### 391 GO BROWN IF YOU'RE FAIR

Black mascara can look too harsh on fair skin and eyes. Instead, plump for brown or brown-black, which will give definition without being startling.

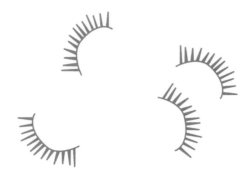

# perfect smile

### 392 GET INTERDENTAL

If you have gappy teeth, bridges or implants, an interdental brush is often better than floss for cleaning between the teeth and keeping gums in the pink.

### 393 GINGER AWAY FUR

If you have a furry tongue, drink more water as dehydration is a major cause of this. If this doesn't work, try sucking on a piece of fresh ginger, which can help reduce bacteria in the mouth naturally.

### 394 BE NATURAL WITH SEAWEED

Seaweed as a food supplement is thought to keep teeth and gums healthy by getting rid of excess plaque, but don't stop brushing and flossing as well.

### 395 CHOOSE CHLORHEXIDINE

Chlorhexidine is the best ingredient to beat inflamed gums or gum disease. It is designed for short-term use and is available in special mouthwashes.

## 396 KISS AWAY YOUR DOUBLE CHIN

It takes 34 individual muscles to pucker up for a goodnight kiss, and the longer it goes on, the better the workout they'll get. Keep cheeks firm with regular kissing, and your partner will thank you, too!

## 397 DISCLOSE YOUR WEAKNESS

Two-thirds of people who brush their teeth twice a day leave plaque deposits behind. Chew a disclosing tablet after brushing and any remaining plaque will turn red, enabling you to spot and target your trouble spots.

## 398 SCRAPE YOUR TONGUE

Tongue scraping is a very important part of oral hygiene as it rids the mouth of bacteria that can lead to bad breath and plaque build-up that can also stain the teeth.

## 399 GET COLOUR CLEVER

To make teeth appear whiter, wear lipsticks in cool, bright hues (pink, raspberry, plum) with a glossy finish.

## 400 JOIN THE JET-SET

Dental water jets are designed to be used after flossing for additional cleaning and polishing. They can be useful for people with bridges, implants or gum disease.

## 401 GUM MASSAGE

Dentists recommend gentle gum massage to strengthen and firm gums, enhance blood flow to the area, fight gingivitis and prevent disease. You can use special gum brushes for this purpose, or massage the gums daily with your index finger – combine with a herbal gum wash or oil for added benefit.

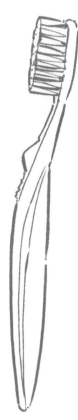

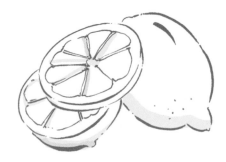

**405 ENLIST YOUR DENTIST**

Use a whitening toothpaste once a week and, more importantly, visit your dentist every six months to have teeth cleaned, especially the gaps between them – it's a sure-fire way of looking more beautiful.

**406 HOME TEETH WHITENING**

Whiten your teeth at home with an over-the-counter gel and tooth tray. You will need to use this for several hours in the day or overnight and should see the maximum results in two or three weeks.

**402 INVEST IN LEMON ZEST**

Whiten teeth naturally by brushing with grated lemon zest, a natural bleaching agent that will whiten teeth without damaging your gums.

**403 SHIFT STAINS WITH STRAWBERRIES**

A simple, natural way to brighten teeth and get rid of stains is to cut a strawberry in half and run the juicy surface along your teeth.

**404 KEEP GUMS IN THE PINK**

Younger gums sit tight on teeth without gaps. To keep gums looking young and healthy avoid over-brushing or brushing too hard, which can contribute to gum recession, making you look older than your years.

**407 LASER AWAY STAINS**

A bleaching system that uses a laser and a whitening gel, is a one-off treatment that gets quick, immediate results. A laser light activates the gel and penetrates the enamel.

### 408 BRIGHTEN YOUR SMILE

Teeth-whitening procedures remove discolouration and staining, up to four shades lighter. Among the various techniques are chemical whitening, mild acid, abrasive, and laser whitening. A clinic procedure is followed by an at-home follow-up treatment. Not suitable for those with sensitive teeth and gums.

### 409 QUICK-TIME ORTHODONTICS

Straight, even teeth can make a huge difference to your appearance. Accelerated orthodontics, a new method, can achieve straightening and overbite or underbite correction in three to eight months, rather than the traditional two or three years.

### 410 VENEER IT WISELY

Veneers, with or without dental re-shaping, can bring uniformity to your smile. Thin porcelain veneers are bonded to your teeth, helping to disguise teeth that are misaligned, worn, chipped or discoloured. They are translucent so light enters through them, making them appear natural.

### 411 SCULPT UNSHAPELY TEETH

There are a variety of options for correcting misshapen teeth, available from dental aesthetics' clinics. Re-sculpting uses gentle abrasion to reshape individual teeth; veneers or laminates are thin porcelain shapes bonded to the teeth.

### 412 PROFIT AND FLOSS

Flossing is one of the most important parts of an oral hygiene routine – use dental floss, tape or wired flossers that can help get to those hard-to-reach areas.

# tools of the trade

### 413 LIGHT IT UP

If you have a habit of overdoing your make-up, make sure you're using a mirror with a powerful enough light. Overdone cheeks or foundation 'tide marks' are common mistakes for people who lack voltage.

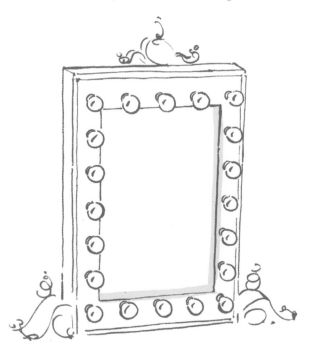

### 414 NO-NO TO NYLON

In most cases use natural bristles rather than nylon or other synthetics, which are stiff and can scratch the face. Most make-up artists prefer natural hair as it blends softly and smoothly.

### 415 GET SHORTY

Most make-up brushes are too long to fit into a small make-up bag. Try getting a travel size version or brushes that twist up from the base.

### 416 SIZE IT UP

For the most effective application, choose make-up brushes that match the size of the area they are to be used on. Brushes for eyelids will be smaller than cheek brushes.

### 417 CULL YOUR MAKE-UP BAG

Make-up might rarely come with use-by dates, but often it's just like food – leave it too long and it will go off. Don't keep lipsticks for more than two years, foundation for more than a year or sunscreen for more than six months to be super-safe.

## 418 LOOK WHERE YOU'RE GOING

Low-level-lighting can completely alter a look. Whatever light you're going to be seen in, try to make-up in a similar light or at least take the time to check how your make-up looks in similar conditions. To avoid mistakes use a make-up mirror that has several light options for day and night and cool and warm lighting.

## 419 KEEP IT DARK AND COOL

Because of the preservatives and active ingredients they contain, all make-up products will last longer and stay more effective if they are kept away from heat sources and direct sunlight. The best place to keep them is in a drawer, fridge or cupboard away from the light.

## 420 BRUSH UP YOUR EYES

Don't be tempted to use fingers to apply eyeshadow – a natural-fibre brush is essential for accurate blending and a professional, well-applied look. Avoid nylon brushes, which will only spread colour around rather than shade the eye.

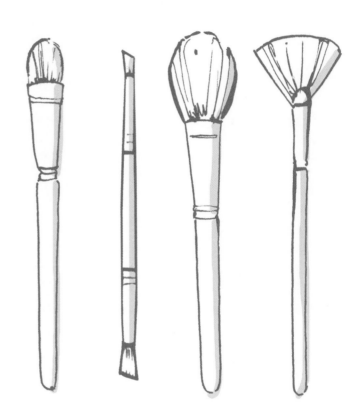

### 421 WATCH FOR COLOUR CHANGES

Throw a product away the moment it starts to change colour, or smells different, as this means the oils have begun to corrupt. If the oils and fats separate, it's a long way out of date, so don't use it.

### 422 FLUFF YOUR LINES

Invest in a large, fluffy brush for applying cheek colour – this will ensure soft, natural-looking lines when you apply it.

### 423 BLEND IT WELL

Everyone needs a blending brush – this should be different from the one you use to apply your eyeshadow, which gets covered in the product. Blending brushes should be soft and clean, and used to give make-up a more natural look.

### 424 WALKING THE THIN LINE

Invest in a thin, flat brush that can be used to apply shaped lines and contours to eyeshadow and highlighter. Use the brush to apply the right amount, then blend with a clean brush to create a professional look.

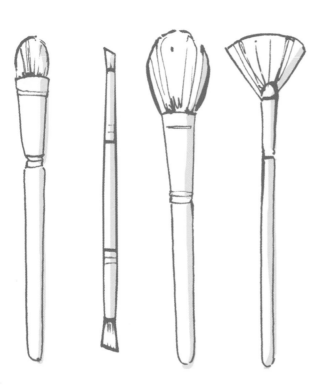

## 425 DON'T GET STUCK IN

Try not to stick your fingers in the pot if you can help it, as this increases the chances of introducing unwanted bacteria into the product. Use a clean, plastic spatula or a spoon instead.

## 426 LAY A GOOD FOUNDATION

Foundation applied with a sponge is a great choice for everyday make-up as it is literally painted onto the skin. The sponge allows you to build-up layers, which means you can start with a thin layer and go thicker for problem areas.

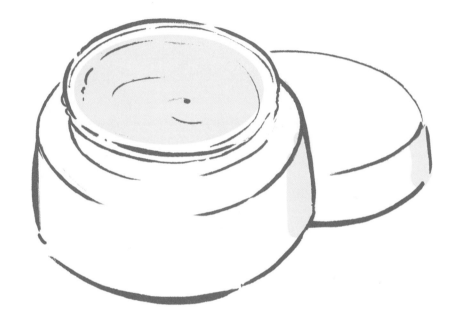

### 427 COLLECT LIKE A PRO

One of the things that sets make-up artists apart is their collection of brushes. Book a make-up lesson and see which brushes they use to do your make-up, then ask them to suggestion an essential at-home kit.

### 428 THE HAPPY MEDIUM

Brushes should not be so stiff that they scratch the face or don't bend against the skin, nor so soft as to be floppy and difficult to control. Medium texture is best.

### 429 VIVE LA DIFFERENCE

There is nothing more frustrating than trying to apply a light shade and getting a darker smudge as a result of the last colour you used with the same brush. Keep brushes for dark and light shades separate.

### 430 MILD BENEFIT

To avoid irritation, use a daily cleanser or a mild washing-up liquid to wash your brushes. These are more gentle alternatives to the specially formulated brush cleaners that can be harsh and cause skin reactions.

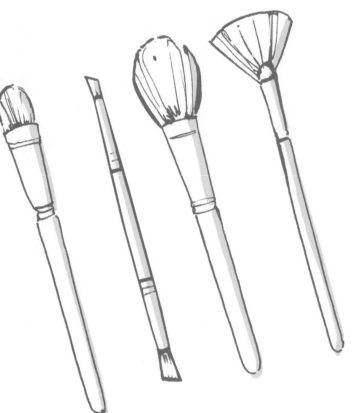

## 431 WASH THOROUGHLY

Wash your make-up brushes in soapy water at least every three months to keep them clean and clog-free. If someone else uses your brushes, wash them thoroughly before you use them again or you risk introducing bacteria into your make-up. Cosmetic sponges and applicators should be washed once a week. Rinse them well and dry flat.

## 432 GET BACK IN SHAPE

Reshape your brushes after washing, laying them out flat and letting them dry naturally before reusing them. If the bristles frizz and shed, it's time to buy new ones as there's no way to recondition the brushes once they are worn out. Keep an eye on the shape, too – each brush has a specific shape for an application purpose and once this deteriorates you will not get good results.

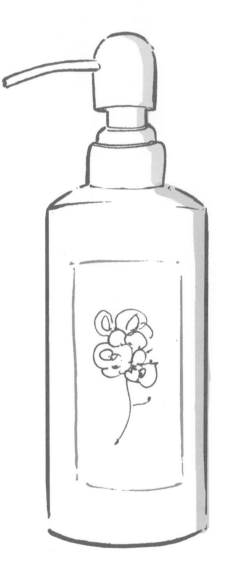

# colour

### 433 A CAP FOR BLONDES

If you have bleached or naturally blonde hair, avoid chlorine, which can make your hair turn green. Cover up with a swimming hat or use anti-chlorine shampoo to keep your colour looking natural.

### 434 HIGH OR LOW LIGHTS?

A highlight lightens and brightens the hair whereas a lowlight darkens and deepens. Highlights are blonde or gold; lowlights can be plum, auburn or chestnut, Usually two or three colours are used throughout for a multifaceted, super-shiny look. Don't go for more than that, or you will scatter the strong effect.

### 435 CARROT JUICE FOR REDHEADS

If you're an orange tone redhead, enhance your natural colour with carrot juice left on the hair for five minutes and shampooed out as normal. The carrot pigment will boost the orange tones and leave your hair looking thick and colour conditioned.

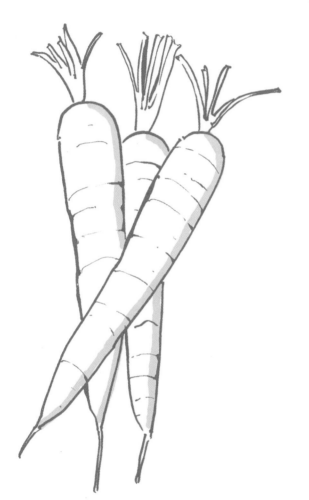

### 436 COLOUR IN THE SEASONS

Get a lift of colour in the late autumn with lowlights. By this time you will have noticed that the ends of your hair are lighter in colour, but also much duller as a lasting result from summer exposure to the sun. A few highlights or lowlights will brighten the hair and act as a winter tonic to perk up your look.

### 437 BEET UP YOUR RED

For a great post-shampoo colour rinse for red-toned hair, infuse a chopped beetroot in hot water for ten minutes and use the water to rinse clean hair through to boost the natural red tones of hair and add depth and richness to colour.

### 438 GET RICH WITH ROSEMARY

To make the most of hair colour, add richness to brunette hair by infusing rosemary in hot water for ten minutes and allow to cool until warm. After shampooing, rinse through with infused water, followed by a small cold-water rinse to add shine.

## 439 COLOUR BLONDE WITH CAMOMILE

A great way to enhance shine and colour in blonde hair is to use cool camomile tea as a rinse following hair washing. This coats the hair and allows the natural blondeness to come through without product build-up.

## 440 BE KIND TO BLEACHED HAIR

If your hair is bleached, use a mild shampoo and the strongest conditioner possible without making your hair go limp, and wash your hair only as often as is necessary to avoid unnecessary drying.

## 441 CAMOUFLAGE GREY HAIRS

Older hair takes colour less well than young hair and skin. Instead of an all-over block colour, try highlights or lowlights, which give hair a sun-kissed appearance without appearing unnatural.

## 442 DO THE DIRTY

Don't turn up at the hair salon for a recolour with freshly washed hair. Roots show up better on unwashed hair, which is also easier to handle.

## 443 BLACK IS NOT FOR BLONDES

Don't be tempted to go too dark in colour if you're naturally blonde. Dark hair tones can flatten out skin and leave you feeling dull as dishwater. If you want to go darker, do it in stages and opt for lowlights rather than all-over colour.

## 444 BE A RINSE PRINCESS

Instead of trying to dye your hair at home, which can lead to unnatural looking results, use a conditioning colour rinse, which will highlight natural colour and help boost the condition of hair as well.

## 445 NO MORE THAN FOUR

Never dye your hair more than four shades darker than its natural colour. It could wash out the colour in your eyes and skin, and leave you feeling pale and pasty.

## 446 GLOVE UP

When dying your own hair, always wear gloves to protect your hands and nails from staining, and apply a layer of moisturizer or Vaseline around the hairline to protect skin.

## 447 SUSTAIN COLOUR WITH SPF

The darker your hair colour, the more important it is to use hair products with SPF protection – sun can bleach away richness, leaving the colour flat and dull.

## 448 PASS ON THE PPDS

If you're going to dye your hair, choose natural vegetable dye rather than dyes containing PPD (Paraphenylenediamine), which can sink into skin and cause health problems. This is particularly important for dark colours, which contain higher levels.

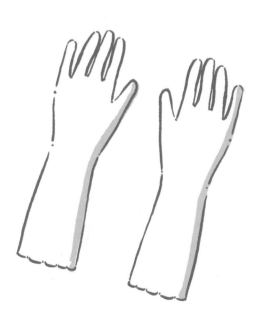

## 449 COLOUR TO MATCH YOUR SKIN

If you have pale skin, avoid hair colours that are too light or white. Instead, go for honey blondes to enhance the natural rose tones of your skin and keep you looking healthy rather than washed out.

## 450 VEG OUT THE GREY

The best way to cover grey hair is to opt for a shade lighter than your own in a natural vegetable dye, which will colour the hair naturally without drying or causing damage.

## 451 AVOID HENNA FOR GREY HAIR

Don't use henna if you want to disguise grey hair because it won't give you a natural colour block – colour will come out redder and brighter on grey hairs, drawing attention to them rather than hiding them away.

## 452 COLOUR FOR VOLUME

Colour boosts volume, giving extra benefit to thin or long hair. However, your volume-boosting shampoo and conditioner may no longer be the right choice if you've coloured your hair. Experiment with different products to see what suits you.

# cut to shape

## 453 HEART YOUR FRINGE

Heart-shaped faces are perfect for fringes –
it will slim down the forehead and
accentuate the bones of the lower face.
Height on top of the head also works, but
beware of long, straight hair or centre
partings that can drag the face down.

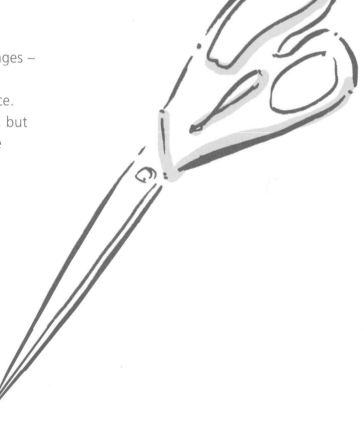

## 454 SEE AN EXPERT

The number one tip for great hair is to get a good haircut. They can be expensive, but you're likely to recoup all the money you've spent on a quality professional because you'll need far fewer products (and time) to make it look good once you get home. The style will keep its shape for longer, too.

## 455 SQUARE UP TO SOFT LAYERS

If you have a square-shaped face, steer clear of bobs or short styles that accentuate your strong jawline. Instead, go for softer layers around the face to break up and cut into the squareness, and bring more attention to eyes and forehead.

## 456 LAYER IT OVAL

Oval faces are the most versatile face shape for styles. They do, however, work best with layers, long or short, which enhance the natural bone structure without lengthening the chin and dragging down the face. Oval faces should avoid blunt fringes and harsh crops.

## 457 SQUARE THE CIRCLE

Round-faced people should avoid fringes and styles that are cropped close or pulled back on the sides of the face. All round fullness is best and crops work well because of the added volume around the face.

## 458 AVOID THE TRIANGLE

If you are growing out hair from a mid to a longer length, you may find that the weight of the hair makes the crown look skull-tight and the ends appear thicker – creating a horrid triangle shape from crown to shoulders. This is flattering to no one, so make sure you get the shape re-cut as it grows to accommodate a style suitable for longer hair.

## 459 GIVE FINE HAIR THE CHOP

Very fine hair should not be grown past the shoulders as it will look thin and weak – if it is blonde it may even seem transparent. Layers and blunt cuts work well, but pay attention to strengthening the hair on the sides of the face where hair is weakest – a fringe may help remedy the problem.

### 460 LAYER IT FULL

Having your hair cut with layers all over, rather than just at the front, will increase the appearance of fullness, making it look larger than life without the need for over-styling.

### 461 GET FRINGE BENEFITS

If you want a change of style without having lots chopped off, ask for a fringe. It will transform your look dramatically. Feathery styles are kinder and easier to maintain than the severe Cleopatra look.

### 462 CHOOSE CAREFULLY

Choose your hairdresser carefully. High-street haircuts can be quite limiting because many chains have specific styles for each season and diversification is discouraged. Make sure your hairdresser is working to make you look your best.

### 463 BE BLUNT

If your hair is thinning or looking fine and wispy, go for blunt ended haircuts rather than feathering. Blunt ends give hair the appearance of being thicker.

### 464 GO SHORTER

Ageing skin and faces ordinarily look better with lighter, shorter haircuts. This is because long hair can 'drag' the face down, making wrinkles appear worse. Also, the shorter your haircut, the more volume it will appear to have.

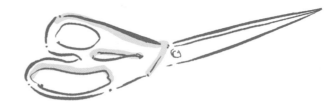

## healthy hair

### 465 PROTECT AGAINST HEAT DAMAGE

Use a thermal protection product before you blow-dry or straighten your hair, especially if you have very curly or afro style hair. The conditioners and polymers in the products will protect your hair.

## 466 SLEEP ON SATIN

Sleeping on a silk pillow can help hair stay smooth overnight because the shaft doesn't stick to it as it does to cotton, leaving it smooth and silky come morning. Wrap a silk scarf around your hotel pillow to keep your holiday hair blooming.

## 467 DO THE TWIST AND SNIP

One temporary method for removing split ends, though not a solution, is to twist a small strand of hair gently until the damaged and split ends appear, sticking out. Holding a pair of scissors vertically, carefully snip off these ends. You will only be trimming the split ends, not the length.

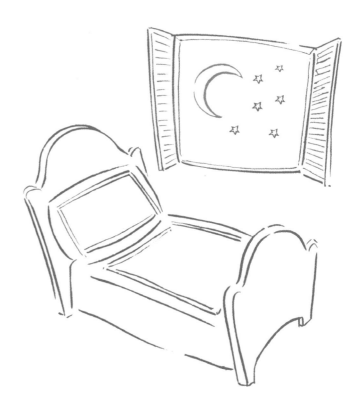

## 468 MEND THE BROKEN SHAFT

Damage to hair, often caused by rough mishandling and using elastic bands that break the hair mid-shaft, can be prevented by taking better care. Do not brush your hair when it's wet, use soft fabric bands or scrunchies to hold your hair back and avoid robust towel drying – instead wrap your hair in a towel and pat and squeeze gently to absorb excess water.

## 469 THICKEN HAIR WITH MASSAGE

One of the signs of ageing is thinning hair. We all lose between 50–100 strands of hair every day but if you're losing more, get a head massage – it will stimulate the roots and help hair growth.

## 470 DETOX DULL HAIR

Use a clarifying shampoo once a week to remove build-up of styling products and accumulated conditioner. Product residue weighs down hair, makes it difficult to style and dulls colour.

## 471 END SPLIT ENDS

Split ends are the bane of anyone with medium to long hair, but they can be prevented by getting regular six-week trims. For an existing problem, use a product formulated for repairing ends. These are applied to the tips of the hair and left in – they won't mend the hair but they will minimize the 'split' appearance. Fortify the hair by using a strengthening shampoo and conditioner.

## 472 AFRO DOES IT

Only use hair products specially formulated for Afro hair – these will not overstrip the hair and will keep the cuticles conditioned and soft. Products with EFA (essential fatty acids) that resemble the natural sebum of the hair will nourish both scalp and hair.

## 473 FLAKE BE GONE

Instead of sticking to an anti-dandruff shampoo all the time, which can be drying, try alternating it with another type of shampoo, so you can help keep your hair in good condition and your dandruff at bay.

## 474 SCOFF SALMON FOR SHINY TRESSES

Salmon is the number one food for shiny, glossy hair. The fish oils it contains plump up the cuticle and keep hair moisturized without being greasy. Other oily fish are good, too – try sardines, anchovies and mackerel.

## 475 DAMAGE LIMITATION

Rather than diet or environment, it is usually mistreatment that causes hair damage. Bleaching, perming, chemical straightening and the overuse of hot appliances all break down the outer cuticle of the hair. The more you indulge in these techniques, the more damaged your hair will be, so limit your exposure. For example, if you lighten your hair, avoid daily use of a blow-dryer or straightener – you can't have it all.

## 476 GROW STRONG AND LONG

Although hair grows only 15 cm (6 in) a year, and you are unlikely to greatly increase this rate, B vitamins, betacarotene and a protein-rich diet may help maximize your growth cycle. Keep your hair one length and always comb from the bottom up, section by section, to avoid breakages.

## 477 DON'T FLAKE OUT

If you suffer from recurrent dandruff or an itchy scalp, try treating your head with tea tree oil, which has been shown to reduce dandruff by up to 40 per cent in sufferers.

## 478 FIX THE FUZZ

Short hairs around the parting and forehead are a sign of damaged new hair growth. Stress or poor nutrition may be to blame, but this could also be a result of directing a blow-dryer at the roots of your hair. To remedy, use a strengthening serum, don't blow-dry near the area and have a deep conditioning treatment in a salon. In the meantime smooth the fuzzy hairs with a conditioning styling cream, not a serum.

## 479 POST-40 HAIR

A sad fact is that after 40, and especially during the menopause, hair thins in diameter and hair growth slows, so we produce less hairs. You may find that changing your haircare regime to avoid harsh products and styling may help redress the problem.

## 480 EAT AWAY HAIR LOSS

Hair loss happens at times of stress and anxiety, often when diet degenerates. Stick to healthy foods like fruit and vegetables to give hair a boost and breathe deeply to replenish oxygen levels.

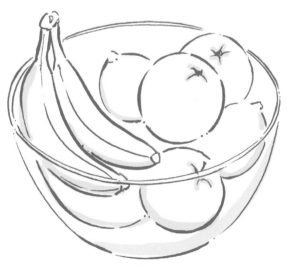

## 481 KELP IT THICK

Sea kelp supplements are thought to help thicken hair with their marine ingredients, which not only promote hair growth and prevent sun and pollution damage, but also add essential micronutrients to the hair root.

## 482 TIE ON A TURBAN

Instead of rubbing hair with a towel, pat it dry instead – wet hair is extremely fragile and rubbing can cause damage to hair shafts. The best way is to wrap hair loosely in a dry towel directly after shampooing to allow the cotton towel to naturally absorb the water. Do not put it on top of the head, which can stretch and knot hair strands, but wrap it along the length, just as it is done in the hair salon.

## 483 DETANGLE FROM THE BOTTOM UP

Trying to detangle knots in the hair from the roots down only results in tearing and stretching of the hair shaft. Instead, start at the bottom and work your way slowly up towards the roots, using a leave-in conditioner to help with difficult areas.

# hair masks

## 484 THICKEN UP WITH WHEAT

To give yourself thick, glossy, catwalk hair and restore flexibility, strength and shine, apply a wheatgerm mask. Soak a little wheatgerm, which is rich in vitamin E, in hot water for five minutes, then drain it and apply the residue to the hair. Leave for five minutes, then rinse thoroughly.

## 485 SHINE UP AN EGG

For flyaway hair, make a homemade conditioning mask to reduce static and add shine by whisking an egg with 200 g (7 oz) of natural (plain) yogurt and massaging into the scalp. Leave for a few minutes, then rinse thoroughly.

## 486 LEAVE IN A HONEY SHINE

For a leave-in treatment that gives extra shine, dissolve a teaspoon of honey into 500 ml (1 pint) of warm water. After shampooing, pour the mixture through the  hair, distributing evenly. Do not rinse out, and dry as normal.

## 487 LIGHTEN UP WITH LEMON

Lemon juice and vinegar are both excellent for oily hair. They will also give lustre to blonde hair and bring out highlights. Never pour vinegar or lemon juice directly onto your hair; dilute them first with water and distribute evenly.

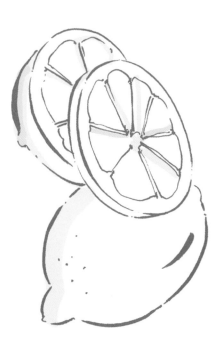

## 488 MOISTURIZE WITH OLIVE OIL

Olive oil is nature's great moisturizer. Give yourself a deep-conditioning hot oil hair wrap by massaging gently warmed olive oil into the hair and scalp, then wrap your head in a warm towel (which has been heated in a tumble dryer briefly) for 10–20 minutes. Follow by shampooing, conditioning and drying as usual.

## 489 COCONUT SHINE

Coconut has long been known for its moisturizing effects. Make your own hair treat by combining coconut oil with a teaspoon of honey for a ten-minute boosting mask that will rescue dry or damaged hair. Those with very dr or curly hair may benefit from massaging the coconut oil into the hair and leaving it on overnight as it naturally softens, conditions and relaxes the hair.

## 490 GET FRUITY FOR EXTRA SHINE

Control oily build-up and add shine with a fruity hair rinse. Heat a sliced orange, a sliced apple and a small slice of melon with 1 litre (2 pints) of water in a saucepan for ten minutes. Strain and allow to cool, then add 500 ml (1 pint) of cider vinegar. Leave for 24 hours before using to rinse hair.

## 491 KEEP YOUR HAIR ON

Tea leaves and lemon juice can be used to prevent hair loss and also help you enhance the natural shine of your hair. Boil and strain tea, then add lemon juice as it cools and use as a conditioner before rinsing thoroughly.

## 492 GIVE YOUR SHAMPOO AN ADDITIVE

Boil a couple of handfuls of mint leaves in 1 litre (2 pints) of water for 20 minutes. Strain and add the mint infusion into a bottle of normal shampoo. Because mint is clarifying, detoxing and cleansing, the infusion is best suited to those with oily-to-normal hair.

## 493 TONE YOUR SCALP

Mix a tablespoon of malt vinegar in a glass of water, and add a pinch of salt. Massage into your scalp with the fingertips and repeat twice a week, leaving on for an hour before rinsing in cold water. The vinegar solution will cleanse and tone the scalp, prevent oiliness and add shine to the hair.

## 494 DIY SHAMPOO MASK

Whisk together equal amounts of castor oil, glycerine, cider vinegar and a mild herbal shampoo. Massage into the hair like a normal shampoo, but leave on for 10–20 minutes before rinsing. The shampoo mask will add shine to dull, lacklustre hair.

# shampoo & condition

### 485 WASH THE ROOTS, NOT THE ENDS

When shampooing, concentrate on the roots, not the ends, of the hair – this will clean the greasiest sebum-producing area without stripping the drier parts. Don't worry about not being clean – the shampoo will cleanse the length of the hair as it rinses out.

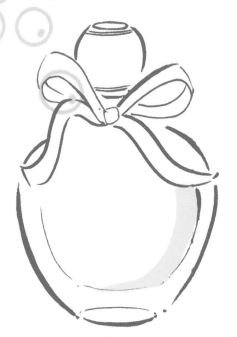

## 496 GET HANDY WITH SHAMPOO

Instead of squeezing shampoo directly onto the top of the head, ensure even coverage by spreading it over your palms first, working it into a light lather and using your fingers to massage it evenly over the scalp.

## 487 WORK OUT KNOTS

Thoroughly detangle your hair before you wash it – wet hair is much more fragile, so brushing it can cause splits and tears.

## 488 COCONUT CONDITION

Massage hair and scalp with coconut oil to lock moisture into the hair shaft and replenish lost lustre with its light, invisible coating. Coconut also helps to protect against sun and heat damage.

## 489 WASH YOUR HAIR

The best way to wash hair extensions is to soak them in cold water to which a capful of very mild shampoo has been added. Swish them around and then rinse in cool water. Let your extensions air-dry naturally and avoid heat products.

## 500 BUY THE BEST

Cheap shampoos are harsh detergents that are not formulated for the specific needs of your hair. They may contain drying alcohols or resins. Choose the best brand you can afford and buy for your needs – coloured, dry, fine, strengthening, and so on. These have ingredients such as antioxidants, vitamins, sun filters and penetrating strengtheners and moisturizers.

## 501 CONDITIONER FOR ALL

All hair needs a conditioner every time you shampoo. For very fine hair, use a light oil-free variety on the ends of the hair only. Stronger hair may need a leave-in conditioner as well as a rinse-out one.

## 502 SAVE YOUR TIME

All standard conditioners stop working after 30 minutes, so do not leave it on for longer in the belief that you will get greater benefits. For a deep condition, buy a separate conditioner or mask for the purpose – these contain moisturizers and vegetable proteins designed to penetrate into the hair shaft.

## 503 PILE ON THE MAYO

Many commercially bought cholesterol hair conditioners contain alcohol, the very thing that dries out hair. Instead of using one of these, massage a handful of mayonnaise into dry hair and wrap in plastic food wrap for ten minutes to boost moisture.

## 504 BANISH BUILD-UP

One of the major causes of problem hair is product build-up, which can be caused by using too much mousse, gel or spray, and not rinsing thoroughly enough. If necessary, shampoo twice to get really clean and always rinse more than you think you need it.

## 505 GET YOUR PRODUCTS RIGHT

Experiment with shampoos and conditioners until you find one that suits your hair and alternate them with another variety every few months to ensure the ingredients are working to their best ability and your hair's not 'getting used' to them.

## 506 BE PREPARED

If you have a big event to prepare for and you're going to be short of time, or your hair will require styling, wash it the night before and it will be more manageable when you come to style it the next day.

## 507 WET IT DOWN

Make sure your hair is completely soaking wet before shampooing. Leave it under the shower for at least a full minute. You will need less shampoo and washing will be much easier.

## 508 CUT DOWN ON SHAMPOO

For the shiniest hair you've ever had, halve the amount of shampoo you use (a dessertspoon full should be enough for all but the longest hair) and double the amount of time you spend rinsing.

## 509 DEEP CONDITION

If your hair is bleached, give yourself a deep-conditioning treatment once a week to preserve as much moisture as possible in the dehydrated hair shaft and prevent bleach damage spreading through the hair.

# 510 SHINE UP WITH BEER

To give hair a really shiny finish and greater manageability, hairdressers recommend rinsing it in beer, which imparts a luscious, rich shine to the hair follicle. Rinse through with water afterwards to avoid smelling like a brewery!

# 511 GET IN A LATHER

Don't worry about overwashing your hair if you do it every day or every other day. According to the experts, the more hair is shampooed, the better it responds to treatments. It is exposed to the same environment as the rest of your body, so needs to be cleaned just as much as your skin.

# styling

## 512 BLOW-DRY LIKE A PRO

For super-sleek hair, use a round radial brush and blow-dryer on damp hair. Comb through a serum or thermal protector, then divide your hair into small, 5 cm (2 in) sections. Work section by section from the nape of the neck to the crown. Place the brush underneath the hair and, directing the nozzle of the hairdryer from the roots to the ends, dry along the length. Move the hairdryer constantly. Be careful not to wrap a big section of hair around the brush, otherwise you could get into a tangly mess. Finish each section with a blast of cold air.

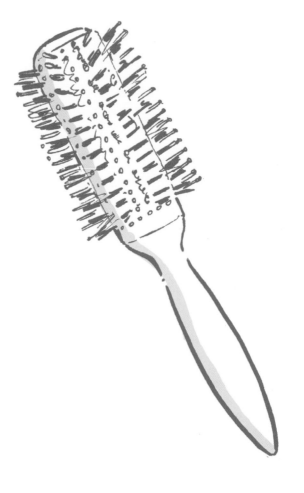

## 513 SELECT SILICONE

A drop of silicone serum will temporarily coat and smooth the hair cuticle and add shine if your hair is frizzy, dry or damaged. Use only a tiny amount to prevent any build-up and concentrate it on the ends if you have fine or greasy hair.

## 514 STAY SMOOTH AND DRY

To dry hair super-straight, use a straightening cream or serum on damp hair. Work down the hair shaft using a hairdryer with a nozzle. If your hair is prone to frizziness, don't dry it upside down or point the airflow upwards, which can roughen up the cuticle – instead, point it down the hair shaft from roots to ends.

## 515 FIGHT THE FRIZZ

If your hair is curly or very prone to frizz, especially in damp weather, try to use a wide-toothed comb, which separates the hairs, rather than a brush. Avoid handling the hair too much and apply serum or a leave-in conditioner with the fingers, smoothing the hair into manageable locks or large ringlets.

## 516 FORESTALL THE FRIZZ

If you suffer from frizzy hair, dry hair completely before leaving the house. Kinking or frizzing can occur if hair is even just a tiny bit damp when you go out in the wind and air.

## 517 KEEP KINKS AWAY

To avoid telltale kinks in long hair do by not put it in a ponytail or bun while it's wet or damp, or for at least six hours after styling if you've used styling products.

## 518 FRENCH PLAIT

For a great way to create waves, especially on thick hair, get a friend to give you a French plait while hair is still damp, then leave it in for several hours and use fingers to tease out the curls.

## 519 ROUGH DRY HAIR BEFORE STYLING

Blow-drying isn't all bad for your hair - instead of blow-drying your hair from wet, rough dry hair until it is 80 per cent dry, then blow-dry or style in sections to avoid heat damage.

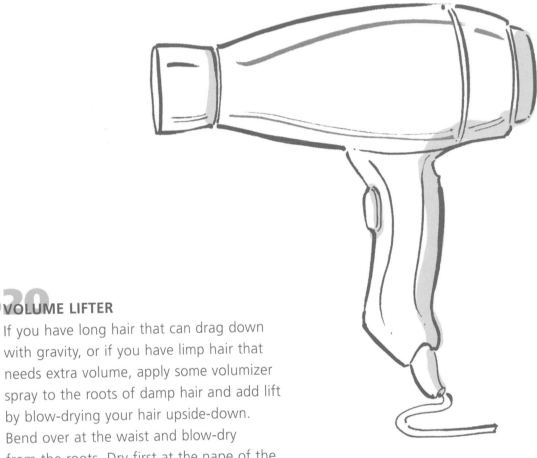

## 520 VOLUME LIFTER

If you have long hair that can drag down
with gravity, or if you have limp hair that
needs extra volume, apply some volumizer
spray to the roots of damp hair and add lift
by blow-drying your hair upside-down.
Bend over at the waist and blow-dry
from the roots. Dry first at the nape of the
neck and finish with the top, front layer.

## 521 MILK THOSE STRAIGHTENERS

According to Indian tradition, milk is an excellent hair straightener. For super-straight hair, spritz milk onto the hair while it's still damp, then let it set for 20 minutes before rinsing and shampooing as usual.

## 522 STOP THE STATIC

To remedy flyaway, static hair, which is especially a problem in hot, dry weather, spray hairspray on your brush and brush through your hair. Alternatively spritz with water. Always use a moisturizing shampoo.

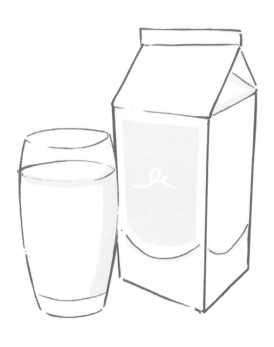

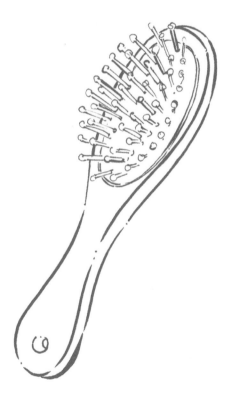

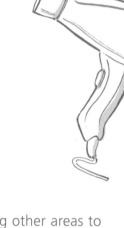

## 523 VOLUMIZE WHILE WET

The most effective way to use volumizing mousse is to apply it to damp hair and then blow it dry – this will help boost body, especially if you concentrate on lifting at the roots. Use a volumizing shampoo and conditioner and a short style with lots of layers will help lift flat, lank hair.

## 524 START AT THE BACK

Apply styling products first to the back of the hair, where you have most hair, working your way forwards to the front sections. This will ensure even distribution and prevent you from adding too much product to the top of the head.

## 525 DRY NATURALLY

Allow hair to dry naturally as often as possible to restore hair health, rather than always reaching for the hairdryer and styling tools. If you hate your frizzy curls, apply a serum and twist large ringlets around your fingers as your hair air-dries – this creates large sleek curls rather than frizzy ones and you may love your new look.

## 526 NOZZLE AWAY FRIZZ

A great way to prevent frizz and flyaway hairs when blow-drying is to use the nozzle attachment of your hairdryer, which will target hair exactly and enable you to dry it in sections without causing other areas to frizz up.

## 527 ROUND IT OUT

For shorter, layered styles, apply mousse and then use a round brush to dry and style the hair. This will add volume and sleekness without curl. Once dry, shape the style with your fingers and finish off the ends with a little wax or gel for added definition.

## 528 GET SILKY SHINE

Smooth silk can boost the natural shine of your hair and help smooth down follicles. Wrap a silk scarf around your hairbrush and 'brush' your hair with it to add lustrous shine.

## 529 EXTEND AWAY

You don't have to splash out on expensive hair extensions to get mermaid-like tresses. Instead, try at-home clip-in hair extensions, which will give you the A-list look without breaking the bank. You will then know whether you'd like to go for the real McCoy or not. Likewise, if you are thinking of changing your cut or colour, try on different wigs so you can experiment first.

## 530 SAY ALOE TO SMOOTH HAIR

If you have curly hair and don't want it to frizz, but would like to keep that natural shine, apply a small amount of aloe vera, which will smooth the hair shaft without weighing it down.

## 531 SOFT FOAM CURLS

Avoid the heat damage of hot rollers by using bendy foam curlers to achieve a smooth ringlet look. Apply a little setting lotion, then wind your hair around the curlers. Leave in overnight and you will have curls you can finger through and break up for a casual look.

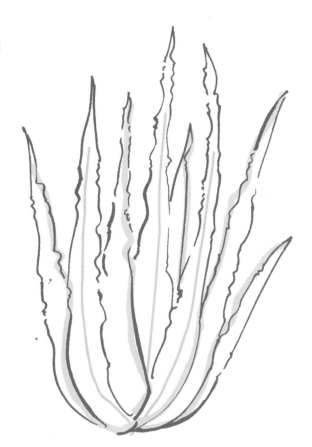

## 532 TRY TOUSLED TRESSES

Instead of leaving hair looking groomed to within an inch of its life, try spraying a mist of volumizing lotion onto it and style with fingers only to add texture and avoid that over-brushed look.

## 533 GET SET TO SHOWER

When using non-heated rollers, put your hair in them before taking a shower and the steam will help set the curls for a longlasting style when you take them out. Make sure you wait until the hair is fully dry before removing the rollers.

## 534 CHOOSE VELCRO FOR FINE HAIR

Velcro rollers provide soft curl and full body, and can be used on either damp or dry hair. They are good choices for short or fine hair and hair that breaks easily, since they don't need to be clipped in place.

## 535 NEW DAY, NEW LOOK

For a new look without a cut, simply change your parting. If you are used to a side parting, a centre one can really make your features stand out and give you a fresher, younger look.

## 536 BE LONGLASTING WITH GEL

Suitable for short, layered or intricate styles that need firm hold, gel will allow you to shape the hair to some extent, keeping it in position. It is best applied either wet and allowed to dry naturally in shape, or after a blow-dry. If you apply it before you blow-dry, you are likely to get an unattractive flaky residue.

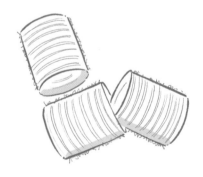

### 537 WAX IT UP

Wax is a great product to add shine and separation to short or medium choppy styles. First, rub wax between the hands to warm it and then distribute it evenly and lightly all over the hair. Do not apply it in pieces to bits here and there as you won't get the full shine benefits.

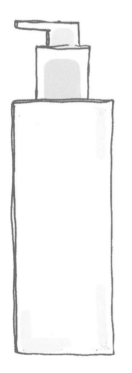

### 538 DON'T HEAT EXTENSIONS

If you want to style or curl acrylic hair extensions, be sure to use rollers with no thermal styling products and take care using hot blow-dryers or other styling tools. Most extensions are not made of real hair and may burn. To prolong the life of your extensions, whether they are natural or acrylic, never sleep with wet hair and do not try to dye them yourself at home – always visit a salon for colour.

### 539 GO LOOSE FOR ROLLERS

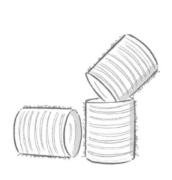

Never wind rollers too tightly, or you could end up with hair loss and damage as the hair is stretched, torn or pulled out from the root. Remember, hair contracts when drying, so if you're putting them on wet hair, give yourself a bit of extra room.

### 540 SHINE ON THE SPRAY

To get instant lustrous shine all over, use a spray gloss in the same way as you would hairspray. This is a gloss product that delivers a fine, light mist without leaving the heavy slickness of a serum.

# styling tools

## 541 DON'T NEGLECT BRUSHES

Just like your hair, your brushes, combs and styling tools need regular washing to maintain tiptop form. Use shampoo or mild detergent to keep them sparkling clean.

## 542 PLACE YOUR ORDER

For medium-length to long hair, you're best off using a chunky, barrelled brush but often these aren't available in shops. Ask your hair stylist to order you one for a professional approach at home.

## 543 GET DRY QUICK

Brushes with holes in the base or around the barrel help the flow of air through the brush and can enable you to dry hair more quickly, boosting volume by targeting all areas of the hair shaft and root.

## 544 DON'T BE CAUGHT WITHOUT A PADDLE

With their large, flat bases, paddle brushes are great for smoothing out medium-length to long hair. If you want to blow-dry your tresses straight and shiny, hold the brush perpendicular to the hair and aim the blow-dryer at the base of the brush.

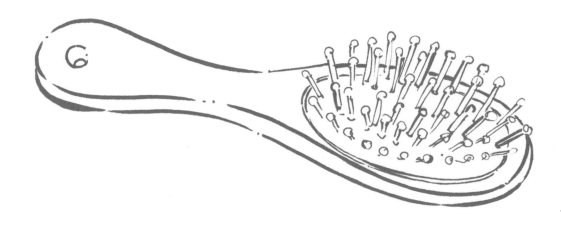

## 545 AVOID EXTREME IRONING

Flattening irons can dry and break the hair if they get too hot or are used too often. Save straighteners for special occasions and for everyday straightening, use a brush that features heat-retaining vents to allow the hot air to pass through. For the best straighteners, choose those with ceramic plates and a ceramic heating element, and avoid wet-to-dry varieties which can damage hair when it is at its most fragile.

## 546 GO WIDE FOR THICK HAIR

Wide-spaced and staggered rows of bristles enable a brush to slip through the hair more easily, which is an important feature if you have thick, wavy or curly hair that tangles easily.

## 547 DON'T KEEP DAMAGED GOODS

When the bristles of your hairbrush start looking damaged, bent or frayed, or the brush starts losing bristles, it's time to replace your hairbrush. Over-used bristles can damage and pull hair, causing split ends and tearing.

## 548 ROLL OUT THE BARREL

Small to medium round or barrelled brushes work best on shorter hair, and for creating flick-ups, while big barrelled brushes are often favoured by hairdressers for blow-drying medium-length to long hair because they hold more hair and won't cause knots. Extricating long hair that has been caught up in too-small barrel brushes will cause pain and tears.

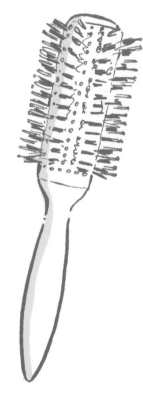

## 549 BUY THE BEST BRISTLES

Avoid hairbrushes with synthetic bristles, which can be harsh on both the hair and the skin of the scalp. Opt for combs or natural fibres instead, such as boar bristles. If you can only afford synthetic varieties, choose ones with round-tipped or ball ends.

# body masks

### 550 LOSE INCHES WITH CLAY

Clay products are great home spa choices for inch loss because they leach excess fluids out of the skin and help tone and tighten skin, especially if used with compressing bandages to squish cells together. The more absorbent the clay, the more inches will be lost.

### 551 REVITALIZE WITH ROSE

Make a revitalizing body mask with rose and lime by mixing rosewater and lime juice with a little glycerine and use the lotion on dry skin after a bath. Store in the fridge if you want to keep it for more than a few days.

### 552 GO NON-GREASY

Create a moisture-boosting, skin-conditioning body mask which won't make skin greasy using witch hazel and olive oil, which will leave skin feeling great without making oily areas oilier. Apply just enough to soak in well.

## 553 PLAY DEAD

Dead sea salts are fantastic for replenishing skin health and boosting circulation. For best results, lie back in a bath and gently massage skin to absorb the salty goodness.

## 554 MAKE YOUR OWN WRAP

The most simple wrap is clay with added salt, which is highly absorbent. Warm some water, add ingredients then dip in bandages and wrap yourself in them. You can add herbs such as rose petals, camomile or ginger powder, if required.

## 555 BOOST CIRCULATION

If you're using a body mask, tighten up problem areas using gently wrapped plastic wrap or bandages, which can improve circulation by tightening the skin and helping it to release toxins.

## 556 GO FOR SEA CLAY

Sea clay is the best detoxifying product to help leach toxins out of the skin and boost circulation in underlying areas. For best results, use bandages or (old) towels to compress it onto the skin.

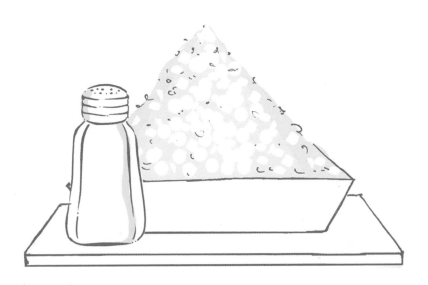

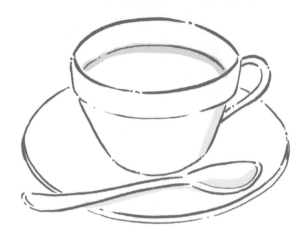

## 557 DON'T DRINK CAFFEINE

If you're having a body wrap, avoid caffeine, fried food, sugar and fizzy drinks for 24 hours before and after the treatment to boost its efficiency. All of these can add to toxin build-up and reduce the treatment's action.

## 558 GO FOR ALL-OVER RELAXATION

Don't forget to make sure you allow yourself time to wind down after a body treatment, as you may feel sleepy, or even dizzy or faint. Listen to your favourite music, read a book or have a cup of herbal tea. Allowing yourself to de-stress will prolong the effects of the experience.

## 559 BATHE BEFOREHAND

If you're using a body mask or wrap at home, take a warm bath or shower beforehand to open pores and make the treatment more efficient at leaching toxins. Similarly, do the same before you visit the spa.

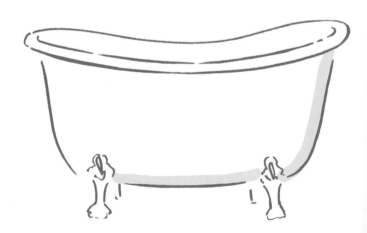

## 560 HOT AND COLD

Bath temperatures can be used therapeutically, but may not achieve the relaxing treat you are looking for. Cold baths reduce swelling by constricting blood vessels while hot ones relieve muscle soreness and eliminate body toxins.

## 561 FLUSH IT OUT

Drink lots of water before, during and after body masks to help remove toxins and stimulate the lymph system. This is especially important for detoxifying treatments, which are very dehydrating.

## 562 DRINK BE WARM

Choose a warm room for body masks and treatments so the mixture stays warm for longer and doesn't dry out. Warmer surroundings boost your circulation, which brings more blood to the surface and helps the mask do its work.

## 563 REST UP

Avoid exercise or anything that makes you sweat for 24 hours after you've had a body treatment or wrap because the sweat could interfere with the ongoing detoxification process. Take gentle exercise if you like but be careful not to overexert.

## 564 MAXIMIZE THE MASK

To maximize the effects of a detoxifying body mask, take a cool or lukewarm bath afterwards and then, two or three days later, take a hot bath which will open up the pores and release any accumulated toxins from the skin.

## 565 WRAP IN THE TUB

To avoid staining your bathroom with clay and other products, stand in the bath to apply your body mask or wrap. You can then easily wash away the excess product without mess.

# cellulite-busters

## 566 STRIDE AWAY CELLULITE

Walking is the best way to reduce cellulite, toning the muscles of the legs, hips and bottom and keeping heart rate gently elevated for fat reduction. Aim for at least 20 minutes brisk walking three or four times a week for best results.

## 567 PEEL OFF ORANGE PEEL

Eating oranges is a great way to reduce cellulite because of their high water content, which helps to plump skin. Other fruits containing high levels of water are also useful – try apples, grapefruit and tropical fruits like mango and pineapple.

## 568 UNDERSTAND ENDERMOLOGIE

Endermologie is a salon-based deep-tissue suction treatment that rolls and pinches fatty tissues to break down subcutaneous fat deposits, toxins and retained water. After a number of sessions, you should notice improvements in the overall texture and appearance of the skin.

## 569 DRY BRUSH DIMPLED SKIN

A favourite three-pronged method for dealing with cellulite is to first eliminate toxins from your diet, such as alcohol, caffeine and processed food, then to break it down by using dry skin brushing and lymphatic drainage massage and, finally, to firm up the skin with a good anti-cellulite tightening serum or body cream.

## 570 GO TO GROUNDS

To reduce cellulite, cut out coffee from your diet, but don't throw the grounds away – instead, use them damp as a super-stimulating rub for areas prone to cellulite, working towards the heart in big strokes.

## 571 GET CAFFEINE TIGHTS

Invest in a pair of tights with added caffeine. The idea is that the temperature causes the release of caffeine microcapsules into the skin, increasing metabolic rate and the burning of fat to reduce cellulite.

## 572 MASSAGE IN DEEPLY

Always massage in a cellulite cream, working from the extremities toward the heart and in circular motions – it's the massaging effect that's as beneficial as the cream.

# fragrance

## 573 WAFT IN THE SCENT

Overdoing scent can be annoying to others, especially those next to you on public transport or at work. To ensure a beautiful, delicate application that's not overpowering, spray the fragrance into the air and walk through it – it will linger on your clothes and hair.

## 574 VIAL IT IN YOUR BAG

Invest in a small vial and decant some from the bottle if you want to carry scent around with you in your handbag, or choose a small travel size. If you take the whole bottle with you, and expose it to light or heat, the scent may go off prematurely.

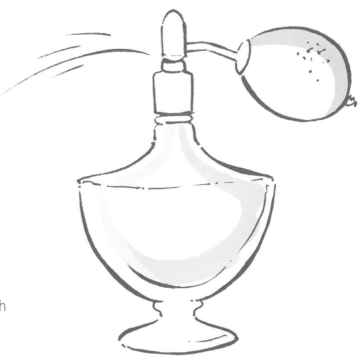

## 575 THROUGH THE WOODS

Chypre scents are based on mossy and fern notes that are often combined with jasmine, rose or citrus, and are ideal if you like warm, aromatic scents.

## 576 KEEP IT BOXED UP

Keeping perfumes in their boxes shields them from light, which can cause chemical changes in their make-up and helps them last longer than if exposed to light.

## 577 BE CONSCIOUS OF COLOUR

Throw your perfume away if it changes colour (especially if it goes darker) or starts to smell different, as this means irreversible changes have taken place in the bottle, which could cause skin reactions.

## 578 GET SCENTS-IBLE

Perfume and scent can change the way you feel. To give yourself a lift, opt for citrus scents or vanilla, and for sexy evenings, try musk or rose.

## 579 DAYTIME FOR FLOWERS AND FRUIT

Traditionally the two fragrance families of florals and citrus are reserved for day. Florals are feminine and easy to wear, ranging from single notes to bouquets that include rose, lily of the valley, freesia and violet. Citrus is crisp, refreshing and tangy.

## 580 TEST ONLY FOUR

Don't try more than four scents at once, however tempting it is when trapped in a department store. You won't be able to differentiate between them, though sniffing coffee will help readjust your 'nose'.

## 581 A WATERFALL OF SCENT

The ozonic family of fragrances has watery notes that are often used to enhance floral, oriental and woody fragrances. If you like the fresh air feel of the seaside, these scents are right for you.

## 582 GET IN A DIFFERENT MOOD

Because most eau de toilettes are potent for only four to five hours, you can change fragrances throughout the day to suit your mood. Not many people have a 'signature' scent they stick to for all occasions.

## 583 DON'T SPRAY ONTO SILK

While it is great to have your fragrance on your clothes and hair, avoid spraying directly onto fabric. Many materials, especially silk, will stain permanently.

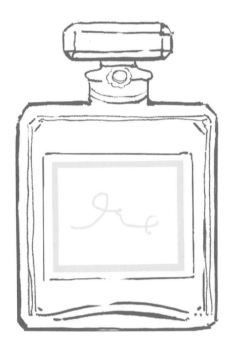

## 584 COOL IS THE RULE

Prolong the shelf-life of your favourite fragrance by keeping it in the fridge. This will help preserve the ingredients, which can often be in delicate balance, and prevent scent changes.

## 585 TRY THIS LOTION NOTION

If your favourite scent doesn't have a matching body lotion, make your own by buying an unperfumed body lotion and adding a few drops of perfume. Make up in small amounts to avoid it going off.

## 586 A FLOWER GARDEN OF SCENTS

Learn to recognize the main flower scent behind the perfume – lily of the valley, one of the most delicate and sweetest flowers, is behind Christian Dior's Diorissimo and Jean Patou's Joy is based on jasmine and rose.

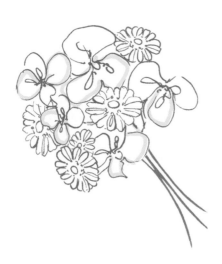

## 587 LIGHT OR HEAVY?

Choose your type of scent according to how you will wear it – eau fraîche only lasts for an hour or two; with eau de toilettes 20 per cent of the scent will last all day; with eau de parfum 30 per cent lasts all day; and with perfume 50 per cent lasts all day.

## 588 MAKE IT LAST

Layer your favourite fragrance to make it more effective by using matching products – the shower gel, body lotion and perfume.

## 589 ORIENTAL FRAGRANCES

Spicy musks, woods and ambers form the basis of this sultry and seductive family of fragrances. They are heavier and longer lasting, making them popular for evening.

## 590 CARE IN THE WORKPLACE

If you love wearing perfumes, be thoughtful of others in the workplace or public spaces. Although you may love the scent, it can be a hazard for others, triggering asthma, migraine and other allergic reactions.

### 591 CHECK YOUR REACTIONS

Perfume is a common cause of allergies and skin reactions, which don't always happen in the exact area of application. If you think this might be the case, try cutting it out for a few days and see if the problem disappears. Avoid wearing any fragrance in the sun as it can cause rashes.

### 592 TAKE A BREAK

There is some evidence that sensitive skins can 'get used' to a fragrance if worn every day, which could lead to skin reactions if you stop using it for a while and then start again. To prevent this problem, don't wear the same scent every day.

### 593 PHONE A FRIEND

If you wear the same scent most of the time, the chances are that your nose has adapted to the smell, which could lead to you using too much. If you've used the same scent for a year or more, ask a close friend to tell you honestly how strong your scent is on a scale of one (negligible) to ten (overpowering).

### 594 WEAR IT NAKED

Don't simply add perfume on your way out the door – it needs the warmth of your skin to interact with the oils. Scent should be worn directly on your skin under your clothes for lasting effect. Put it on pulse points low on the body as it will rise with your body heat. Be like Marilyn Monroe and only wear Chanel No. 5 to bed!

### 595 A NOSE FOR NEW SCENTS

When trying out a new scent, wait up to five hours for it to develop on your skin – this way you will first smell the top notes, then the middle at about 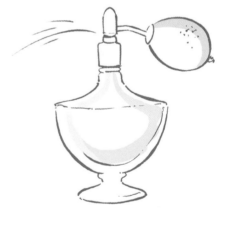 two to four hours later (the important notes) and finally the full base note.

# hair removal

## 586 TRY TURMERIC

The best natural depilatory is a turmeric paste, which gets rid of even thick hairs. Apply it before a bath, and leave it on to dry, then simply wash off for a naturally smooth look.

## 597 WARM UP INGROWING HAIRS

For ingrown pubic hairs along the bikini line, hold a hot compress against ingrown spots for ten minutes a couple of times a day to soften the skin and help the hairs work their way out.

## 598 POINT TO THE PROBLEM

Ingrown hairs on your bikini line, underarms or legs can be gently removed with a pair of pointed tweezers.

## 599 DON'T OVERSOAK

Try not to soak in the bath too long before shaving or run the water too hot, as this causes skin to wrinkle and swell slightly, making a close, clean shave more difficult.

## 600 CALM DOWN WITH CAMOMILE

Many spas use camomile wax, which is normal wax infused with calming camomile, which can ease pain and redness following waxing. If you have sensitive skin, this can mean happier hair removal – ask your beautician for advice.

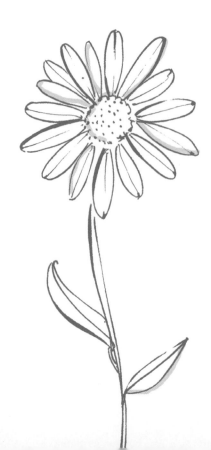

## 601 A SUGAR SOLUTION

Sugaring is often a better choice than waxing if you have somewhere to go afterwards, as wax can stick to legs but the sugar solution is water soluble, which means it wipes off, leaving no telltale marks. Sugar waxing works in exactly the same way as traditional waxing but because the solution is sugar-based, it dissolves in water, so there is no sticky residue to clean from your skin.

## 602 EXFOLIATE BEFORE YOU WAX

To avoid ingrown hairs post-waxing, remove dead skin cells, which might obstruct the hair beforehand by exfoliating the area to be waxed. Because skin will be softer, you are less likely to develop ingrown hairs.

## 603 BLEACH AWAY DOWN

If you have downy hair on your forehead or in front of your ears, rub a freshly cut lemon over the hair and leave for five to ten minutes before rinsing off for a natural bleaching agent which won't make them bright white.

## 604 WAIT AND SEE

If you have ingrown pubic hairs, don't be tempted to overexfoliate as this could cause further skin trauma, which may result in sore spots, infections or more serious irritation of the skin. Wait until it's gone and then exfoliate.

## 605 SHAKE AND WAX

When waxing your hair at home, first shake talcum powder over the area to be waxed as this helps the strip to rip and be more effective.

## 606 DON'T RUB RED SPOTS

If you have red spots caused by ingrown hairs or sore patches following hair removal on your bikini line, wear loose-fitting underwear and clothing until the bumps are gone to avoid friction.

## 607 POP A PILL

If you find the pain of waxing or epilating too much to bear, lessen the pain by taking paracetamol or ibuprofen 15 minutes beforehand to help reduce your suffering.

## 608 GET IT ALL OUT

When waxing, sugaring or plucking, be sure to pull the hair out by the roots by pulling in the direction of hair growth in smooth, even pulls. Do not allow the hair to break below the skin surface, which can lead to rough regrowth and ingrown hairs.

## 609 TO POINT OR ANGLE?

If you're plucking areas like the eyebrow, chin or upper lip, choose angled tweezers for targeted hair removal – the slant makes it easier to grasp and pluck in the direction of hair growth, which reduces soreness and redness. Pointed tweezers should be used to extract very short hairs.

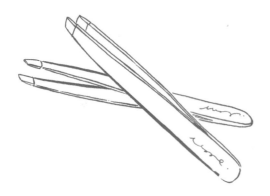

## 610 GO FLAT FOR LARGE

For large areas of hair removal, such as touching up patches on legs or arms which have been missed with waxing, use flat-headed tweezers, which can pull more than one hair out at a time and make plucking more efficient and quicker. Remember to always pluck in the direction of hair growth, so make sure the hairs are all growing in the same direction.

## 611 BEWARE OF WAXING

If you are using Retin-A, Accutane or other skin-exfoliating medications, you should tell your beautician before your waxing appointment as this can cause increased skin sensitivity. The therapist may decide to modify the treatment accordingly.

## 612 DON'T WAX ON SUNBURN

Laser peels and sunburn are two big no-nos for waxing. Because both procedures expose the more sensitive layers of the skin and can cause redness and heat retention in skin layers, you should avoid waxing within a week of either of them.

## 613 CONDITION AND SHAVE

If you have run out of shaving foam, use hair conditioner when shaving legs. Because it's smooth, it will stop the skin dragging and help you shave smoothly without stretching the skin.

## 614 KEEP IT TO YOURSELF

Never be tempted to use someone else's razor or let them use yours. It could open you up to the chances of infection because it's so close to the skin's surface and ther the risk of cutting and nicking skin.

## 615 BE A WATER BABY

To ensure an extremely close shave, soften hairs first by having a short, warm bath as this is a great way to hydrate before shaving and hair is easier to cut when wet and supple.

## 616 REDUCE FACIAL HAIR WITH ROSE

Stimulating facial hair will cause it to grow more. To keep it unstimulated, use a light toner like rosewater and a light moisturizer that won't nourish the hair root.

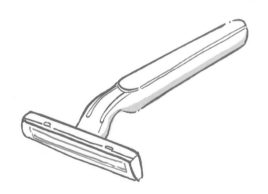

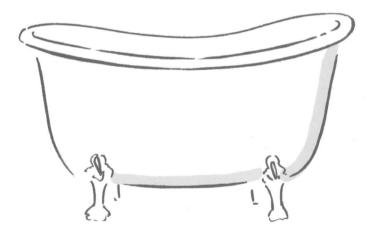

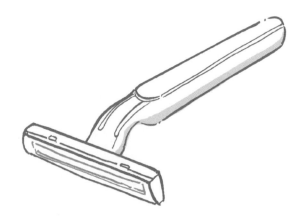

### 617 WET SHAVE FOR SMOOTH SKIN

As any barber will tell you, wet shaves are the most effective. Before shaving, wet the hair as well as the skin, use a foam or mousse specifically for shaving, and pull the skin taut to ensure a smooth finish. Work upwards with long, even strokes.

### 618 TAKE IT ON THE SHIN

The skin on the shin is especially thin and prone to becoming dry, wrinkled and flaky if neglected, so pay special attention when shaving this area and slather on a moisturizer every morning, through the whole year, to keep legs smooth.

### 619 AVOID THE TIME OF THE MONTH

In the few days before your period, when hormone levels in the body are out of balance, waxing can be more painful then at other times of the month, so check your diary before you de-fuzz.

### 620 KEEP YOUR COOL

Avoid saunas, hot baths, exercise or sunbathing for 24 hours after waxing. All of these can raise your body temperature, which means you may sweat more, causing irritation to treated areas.

### 621 LASER HAIRS AWAY

A new treatment for permanent hair loss, laser removal is most effective where there is high contract between the hair and skin, such as dark-haired people with pale skin.

### 622 GET TRIM

Trimming hair with nail scissors before waxing makes the job a lot easier, avoids tangles and can reduce pain. You'll also be able to make sure you get straight lines to avoid that uneven look.

# hands & feet

### 623 TAKE OUT TOBACCO STAINS

Rub tobacco-stained fingers and nails with half a freshly cut lemon for five to ten minutes to help bleach skin naturally without drying it out. Rubbing the back of the hands with lemon will also fade age spots.

### 624 SUN-PROTECT YOUR HANDS

In summer, add a layer of sunscreen to your hands or use a hand cream with SPF to protect skin against dryness, wrinkles and premature ageing.

### 625 SCRUB WELL

Mix a paste of almond oil and salt in the palm of one hand and use to scrub the back of your hands and over your knuckles – your hands will feel and look silky smooth.

### 626 GO HAND IN GLOVE

Prevent problems by wearing rubber gloves when washing dishes and doing other household chores. Keep exposure to harsh chemicals, especially bleach, to a minimum.

### 627 BOWL HANDS OVER

For hands that are smooth and wrinkle free, soak them in a bowl of warm water for five minutes before drying and applying your favourite hand cream. The water soaks into the skin and the cream forms a barrier, locking it in and easing aches and pains at the same time.

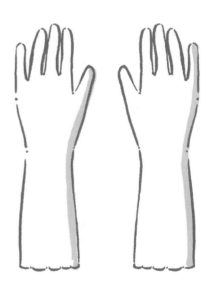

135

## 629 GET SOME WRIST ACTION

To ease tired hands and give yourself a circulation boost, hold both hands in front of you with palms facing inwards, loosen their wrist grip and flap them backwards and forwards. Feel them tingle as the blood rushes to them.

## 630 KNOW THE BACK OF YOUR HAND

The skin on the back of your hand is an excellent way to test for dehydration. Pinch it and count how long it takes to return to being smooth. If it's more than a second, your skin's telling you it needs a drink.

## 631 GIVE A TIGHT SQUEEZE

If you have dry finger ends, hang nails or flaky, ridged nails, give them a boost by squeezing the tip of each finger as hard as possible for about five seconds to activate blood circulation into the nail bed.

## 632 KEEP CREAM TO HAND

Do as all the beauty editors do and keep hand cream by all your taps (faucets) so it's easy to reapply cream whenever you wash.

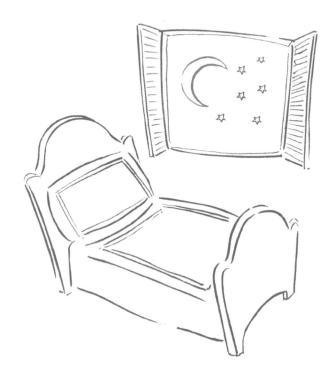

## 628 SLEEP ON THE JOB

For an overnight treat for hands that will moisturize and firm skin, slather on a generous layer of rich hand cream, then put on a pair of gloves and leave overnight.

## 633 STAY OUT OF HOT WATER

The repeated use of soap and water damages the top layer of the skin and can cause chapping. Avoid strong soap and hot air dryers, and opt for lukewarm water rather than the hot tap alone.

## 634 KEEP HANDS YOUNG

Take care of your hands before they give away your secrets. Hand skin is frequently neglected, but it's often the real telltale sign of age. Invest in a rich hand cream day and night to keep your hands looking young and tender.

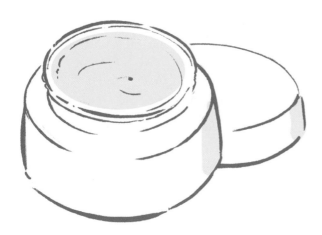

## 635 SALT AWAY STIFFNESS

If you have stiff, sore or aching hands, soak them in salt water for 15–20 minutes, then rinse with fresh water. This will help reduce swelling and restore the fluid balance.

## 636 BAN WARTS WITH DANDELION

Dandelion stems have long been believed to help banish warts. Apply the juice of a dandelion stem two or three times daily for several weeks.

## 637 BE A BAREFOOT BEAUTY

Allow feet to breathe and you'll avoid many unsightly problems like fungal infections. Use natural, breathable fibres whenever possible for socks and try to go barefoot for at least an hour a day.

## 638 TREAT ATHLETE'S FOOT WITH TEA TREE

Tea tree oil, with its naturally astringent and antibacterial properties, can help prevent the spread of athlete's foot by drying out skin and making it hard for the fungus to spread.

137

## 639 ORANGE IS THE AGENT

Massage feet with orange oil, which will help draw out toxins and impurities from the skin and boost the regeneration of cells. Rub the ball of the foot in a circular motion, and work your way down the sides to the heel.

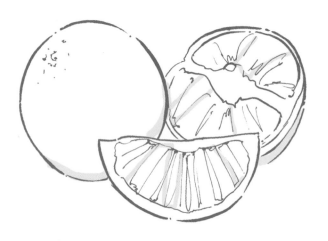

## 640 COOL WITH MANGO

Cool hot, burning or swollen feet with mango juice, which rejuvenates skin as well as reducing the pain and discomfort of problem feet. Soak feet for a few minutes or apply with cotton wool before a warm bath.

## 641 GET FEET FIT

Keep feet and toes flexible by standing and walking on tiptoe whenever you can. And practise picking up pencils or marbles with your toes.

## 642 SOCK IT TO DRY FEET

Before bed, exfoliate feet and rub in cream or oil, then pull on a pair of socks to help them make the most of their newfound moisture all night long. When you wake up, they'll be as soft as a baby's!

## 643 NEVER SHARE SHOES

Other people's shoes, especially if they're well worn favourites, will have moulded to their feet, which could cause you problems if you borrow them by putting pressure on areas which might not be used to it.

### 644 PEP UP WITH PEPPERMINT

Invigorate the tired skin of your feet and lower legs with products infused with essential oils of peppermint and eucalyptus, which have been shown to have revitalizing effects. Or choose an unscented product and add your own.

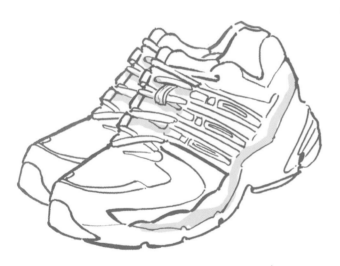

### 645 PUMICE AWAY HARD SKIN

To remove hard skin on feet, rub with a pumice after soaking the feet for at least ten minutes to soften problem areas, such as the balls of the feet and the heels. The natural stone will not only remove dead skin but will boost circulation to the area, encouraging regeneration.

### 646 WEAR THE RIGHT SHOE SIZE

Squeezing your feet into too-small shoes can cause longterm problems as corns and callouses build-up on pressured areas and areas of dry skin mount up to help protect the feet against shoe pressure. Fit and buy shoes in the afternoon when your feet are the most swollen and remember that air travel and pregnancy will make feet swell.

### 647 CHANGE IT AROUND

Don't wear the same shoes for more than a few days running, because your feet will begin to adapt to wearing them and you may get problems in pressured areas. Switch between flats and heels, and round and pointed toes regularly.

## 648 SEE YOUR PODIATRIST

If you're suffering corns or callouses, see a podiatrist, also called a chiropodist, who is skilled in dealing with all kinds of foot problems, from verrucas to deformities, and will do more than a pedicurist to help you solve these problems. They will also assess how you walk and the shape of your foot to see if there are any physical reasons for the cause of your problems, and be able to advise and provide surgery for persistent ingrown nails.

## 649 DON'T RAZOR IT OFF

Never remove hard skin with a razor blade, or allow nail technicians or pedicurists to use one on you. This will only spur the skin into producing harder skin to repla it, which defeats the purpose having it removed. Your thera a strong exfoliator scrub or so in the removal of tough skin.

# home spa

## 650 STEAM ROOM

Create your own steam room by closing the door and window in your bathroom and turning on the shower. Your skin will be warmed and primed for further treatment, such as pumicing, pedicures and manicures or body and hair masks.

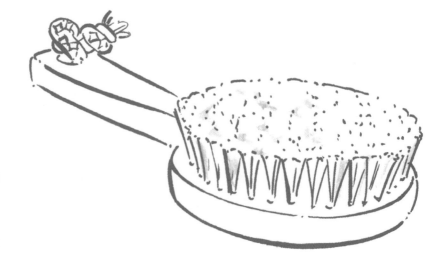

## 651 BOOST BATHING WITH EPSOM

When Epsom salts (aka magnesium sulphate) are absorbed through the skin in a bath, they help to draw toxins from the body, reduce swelling and relax muscles as the skin cools afterwards. Mix a handful of Epsom salts with a handful of sea salt and a splash of bath oil or olive oil.

## 652 WAX IN MOISTURE

Give yourself a home wax pedicure by melting paraffin wax in the microwave to create a wax bath. Moisturize feet well and dip into the wax three times, allowing each layer to dry. The wax should feel warm but not hot. Set for 20 minutes and peel off.

## 653 COMPRESS STRESS

Make a quick stress-relieving compress by adding a few drops of lavender or camomile essential oil to a bowl of warm water and soaking a cotton cloth in it for five minutes, then applying to face and neck as a compress and breathing deeply. Repeat three times.

## 654 PAMPER WITH PATCHOULI

Add a few drops of essential oils to a cup of hot water while you bathe to infuse the room with healing properties. Choose patchouli for lifting the spirits or neroli and ylang-ylang for re-balancing.

## 655 GET SPOTLESS WITH A SPONGE

For the best, non-traumatic face cleansing experience, choose a small natural sea sponge and use small circular motions to work softly over the skin of the face and neck. This will ensure thorough washing without cleansing. Natural sea sponges are softer and last longer than synthetic versions and they don't absorb odour.

## 656 REJUVENATE WITH JUNIPER

If you want a home spa experience to stimulate your circulation and invigorate tired muscles and minds, try adding essential oils of basil and juniper to your bathing experience. They have been shown to have stimulating effects and can pep you up for a good start to the day or right before an important meeting.

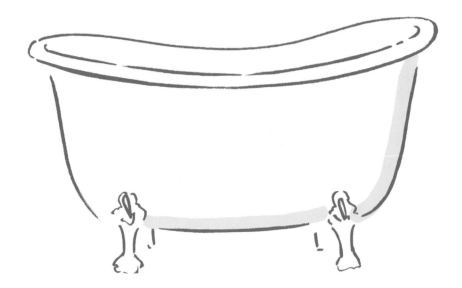

## 657 SOME LIKE IT NOT HOT

For a relaxing bath, make sure the water is pleasantly warm rather than hot, which can stimulate your system and cause the skin to slacken and dehydrate as a result. Always test the water before you enter.

## 658 HAVE A HOME VISIT

Many beauty therapists and stylists will visit your home to deliver a personal and private haircut, manicure or other beauty treatment, bringing all their own equipment, including a massage bed.

## 659 GET A GOMMAGE

For a home spa gommage (salt glow) as good as any salon, mix ground sea salt with 12 drops of a stimulating essential oil such as grapefruit, lemon or thyme. Make a paste by adding enough water to spread easily and apply in brisk circular strokes, especially on hips and thighs.

## 660 TRY CYROTHERAPY

Steal a salon secret (cyrotherapy is extreme cold applied for therapeutic purposes) for your own home – after applying a face-firming treatment, place an ice cube inside a small plastic bag and gently rub over the face and eye area for several minutes to plump up and tone the skin.

## 661 SCENT-SATIONAL PLEASURE

An essential oil diffuser will add to the overall effect of the at-home spa experience. Choose either a relaxing oil such as lavender or an invigorating one like rosemary, according to your mood. Play a CD of nature sounds, turn off all phones and retreat from the world for a few hours.

## 662 GLISTEN WITH GLYCERINE

For a home treatment for dry skin, mix glycerine with lemon juice and use as a moisturizer or face mask to smooth out lines and plump up dehydrated areas.

## 663 COPY CLEOPATRA

Cleopatra was famous for her smooth skin and milk baths. Follow her beauty secret by adding 3 cups of powdered milk or fresh milk to a warm bath. The lactic acid in the milk will soften and gently exfoliate skin.

## 664 GARDEN HERB SOAK

Place a bunch of garden herbs such as rose, lavender and rosemary in a tea strainer and hang it from the running tap in your bath for a healing soak from your own botanical garden!

## 665 LIVE THE FANTASY

Lie back in the tub and float away with a fantasy that you are somewhere exotic. Visualizations like this have been shown to help relaxation by releasing feel-good chemicals in the bloodstream.

# luscious legs

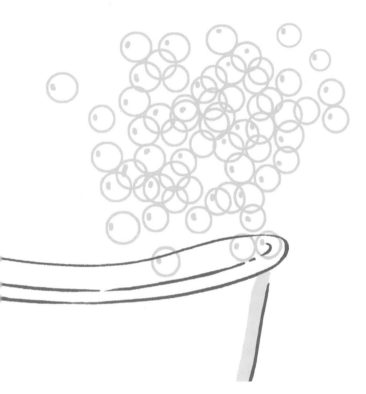

### 667 GO CITRUS FOR VARICOSE VEINS

To reduce the appearance of varicose veins, add extra citrus fruits, grapes, cherries and apricots to your diet. If eaten regularly, these foods can help improve the elasticity of blood vessels.

### 668 SPARKLE AT SOIREES

Don't limit make-up to your face and décolletage. Add some glamorous sparkle to your arms and legs for a sexy evening look. Add a little gold highlighter to your moisturizer and smooth down shins and across shoulder and collarbones to give them shape and shimmer.

### 666 BUBBLE BATH

Many bubble baths and foams can be extremely drying, so if you are planning to have a long soak, make sure the formula includes softening oils in the ingredients list, or else add an oil, such as sweet almond oil, to a ready-prepared solution for extra-moisturizing results.

### 669 GET SMOOTH

For an instant lift to the legs, de-fuzz. Smooth legs look more shapely than hairy ones because the hair can visually reduce the skin's lines and make them appear bigger, especially from a distance. To have thin pins, wax, shave or use a depilation cream regularly and moisturize afterwards.

## 670 BRONZE UP

For a quick fix to make your legs glow, use a body brush to rub off dead skin and then apply a moisturizer with a bronzing pigment to give them a healthy glow in just five minutes, or use normal moisturizer followed by bronzing powder or gel.

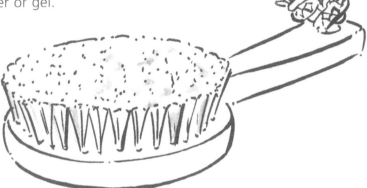

## 671 HOLD 'EM HIGH

To improve the skin and tone of your lower leg, try to get your feet above your head for at least ten minutes a day to improve the circulation and blood flow. Lie on the floor with your feet on a chair, stretch out on the sofa with your feet propped up on the arm when watching television, or even sneak a nap on the bed with your feet up on a couple of pillows.

## 672 GO ROUND IN CIRCLES

Always apply your moisturizer or body scrub in a circular motion from the ankle up as this boosts the circulation of the blood in the legs, facilitating lymphatic drainage and boosting circulation and, therefore, skin health.

## 673 BOOST CIRCULATION

Sometimes, 'big looking' legs may not be fat, but appear heavy because of bad circulation. Put your legs and feet up above hip level for half an hour a day to help fluid flow. If you suffer from varicose veins, this will also help reduce the strain on blood vessels.

## 674 JET LEGS WITH COLD WATER

Finish your shower with a jet of cold water aimed at your lower legs. Not only will this stimulate skin, but it will help constrict the blood vessels in the area, too, boosting the overall appearance.

## 675 AVOID CROSSED LEGS

To reduce swelling in ankles, feet and toes and to prevent the appearance of varicose veins, train yourself not to sit with crossed legs, as this can put strain on blood and lymph vessels and encourage fluid to build up.

## 676 STEP IT UP

There's no better way to give yourself shapely calves than walking up and down stairs. Ban yourself from using elevators or escalators for a month and you'll see visible differences.

# massage

## 677 TOOL UP

Use wooden or plastic self-massage tools, such as balls, rollers and bongers, while you're in the bath to promote relaxation. The added benefit of the warm water helps to make massage more effective, especially if you're trying to unknot tense muscles.

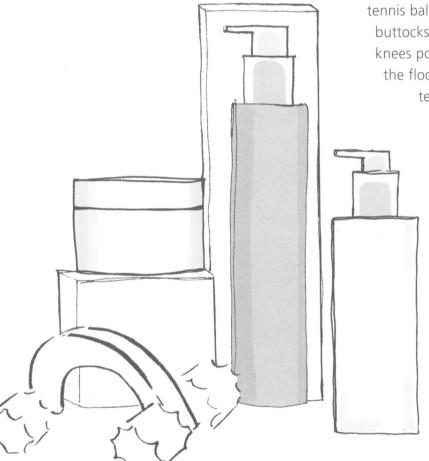

### 678 BE A TENNIS PRO

Instead of shelling out for an expensive salon massage, make your own back relaxer by lying on your back on a couple of used tennis balls, positioned at the top of your buttocks or your lower back with your knees pointing up and your feet flat on the floor. Then roll around to release tension in the back area.

### 679 GET YOUR HAND IN

Give yourself a circulation mini-boost when applying hand cream by using small, circular movements to rub the cream into your knuckles and joints. Use your thumbs to massage the backs of your hands.

## 680 KNEAD BETWEEN THE LINES

Reduce forehead lines caused by tension by using a soft, shallow pinch to relax muscles. Make your hand into a fist, then pinch skin between your thumb and index finger for gentle stimulation.

## 681 BREAST UPLIFT

The thin skin on your breasts is prone to sagging and toxin build-up. Massage problems away using almond oil and gentle sweeping strokes from the underside up into your armpits.

## 682 MAKE THE MOST OF OIL

Use oil during massage to avoid dragging skin and causing it to sag and stretch. Small amounts applied first to the hands are best, as that will ensure you don't use too much.

## 683 SIT UP FOR A GREAT FACE

For facial massages, sit upright or recline rather than stand or lie flat on your back. This will help you breathe evenly and deeply and keep muscles relaxed.

## 684 FINISH WITH A BATH

After your massage, soak in a bath for a ten-minute relaxation. Aromatherapy oils are particularly beneficial at this time because you will already be relaxed and have stimulated skin, which will make the oils more efficient.

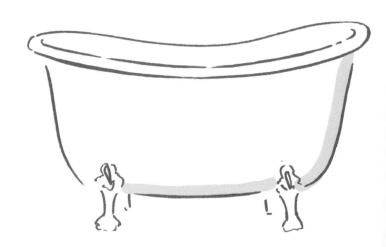

## 685 NURTURE YOUR NECK

With your right hand, gently massage the left side of your neck at the shoulder in a rhythmic motion, working from the base to the ear, and moving slightly round to the back as you do so, in circular strokes. Repeat on the right side of the neck using your left hand. Finish with the fingers of both hands working the back of your neck.

## 686 LIFT THE LID

Droopy eyes can be caused by weak muscle tone in the upper eyelid. Gently massage the surrounding area between your lids and your brows, and along your temples, for a few minutes once a day to improve muscle tone and circulation.

## 687 TAKE THE PINCH

Stimulate circulation in your facial skin by pinching the jawline. Start at the chin, pinching with your thumbs underneath and your fingers on top, and holding for ten seconds. Move along the lower jawbone until you reach the earlobes. Aim for four to five pinches to cover the area.

## 688 CONSIDER THE SINUS POINTS

Massaging the sinus points helps reduce frownlines and facial tension around the eyes. Using the balls of your thumbs or index fingers, apply pressure to either side of the top of your nose for a few seconds. Gradually work down to the nostrils, concentrating on the cartilage at the edge of your nose.

## 689 PAMPER YOUR PEEPERS

Reduce eye strain and wrinkles caused by squinting with a regenerating eye massage. Work fingers along the orbital bone around your eye sockets. Start at the outer edge and work backwards and forwards from the bridge of your nose at least three times.

## 690 GET IN CHEEKY CONDITION

Boost cheek tautness with a quick circulation-boosting massage. Work under the cheekbones with two fingers of each hand, pressing gently, from the middle of your face to the top of your ears, then work back to the middle.

# nails

### 691 MAXIMIZE NAIL GROWTH

To stimulate nail growth, massage the base of the nails with cuticle oil several times a day. This will stimulate and nourish the nail bed, encouraging new growth.

### 692 HEAT UP YOUR NAILS

Bend the fingers of the hands in towards the palms and rub the nails for a minute to give your nails a boost of oxygen and nutrient-rich blood, which will reduce nail problems.

### 693 AIM FOR A PERFECT 10

Don't assume your nine perfect nails will hide the chipped one. If it's small, fill in the chip with a quick coating of colour but if larger re-do the colour on the whole nail.

### 694 CARRY IT OFF

Carry your nail polish with you so you can touch up nails if they chip en route. If this sounds too high maintenance, use a clear shade of gloss, which, if it chips, won't show.

### 695 EXTEND YOUR RANGE

If you have difficulty growing all your nails to the same length, fake it with extensions. Gel versions are glued onto the real nail, then cut and shaped. These are less irritating than acrylic versions, which are longer lasting and stronger but more difficult to remove.

### 696 GO SOFT, NOT LOOSE

The excessive use of nail hardeners that contain formaldehyde can cause lots of nail problems, including peeling, splitting and loose nails, when the nail plate separates from the nail bed. If you suspect this is the source of your problems, go easy on products and use a perfume-free nail cream.

### 697 HANG TEN

If the nails are frequently immersed in water, the outer skin layer may split away from the cuticle causing painful splits or hangnails. Snip off with clean scissors, or prevent problems from occurring by keeping the skin soft with regular applications of moisturizing hand cream.

## 698 PRIME NAILS WITH PROTEIN

When nails easily crack or break they can be a permanent worry. Weak nails may be caused by a protein deficiency in the diet. Increase nutritional intake by eating more lean meat, fish, fresh fruit and vegetables and use a nail cream to help hydrate.

## 699 MEND A BROKEN NAIL

Nail patches are tiny adhesive strips that bring the two sides of a split back together again. They are best applied by a professional manicurist, though there are over-the-counter versions.

## 700 SILK FOR STRENGTH

For nails that repeatedly break or are soft, visit a salon for a silk-wrapping treatment. A thin layer of silk is glued to the nails and buffed into an invisible finish.

## 701 FILE FIRST

For at-home manicures, file first before you remove old nail varnish. The polish keeps the nail protected and if you use a remover first, the nail will be weakened and softer.

## 702 BASE, COLOUR AND TOP

Always follow the three-step programme to varnish your nails: first apply a base coat to protect the nail from discolouring, then apply two coats of the colour, and finish with a clear, glossy top coat for extra shine and to guard against chips.

## 703 DO THE DIP TIP

To speed up nail varnish drying, run nails under cold water for ten minutes to help the varnish form a hard, knock-free coating in no time at all.

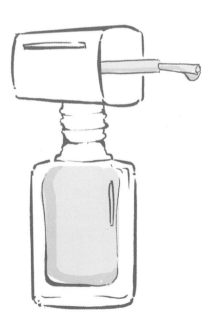

## 704 BREAK FREE OF BRITTLE NAILS

Brittle nails can be caused by over-exposure to the sun, a poor diet or the prolonged use of commercial nail hardeners. Avoid the use of hardeners or varnishes containing formaldehyde, which has a drying effect on nails.

## 705 NICE GIRLS DON'T BITE

To help you stop biting your nails, visit a nail bar each week or every other week. When your nails are nicely filed and varnished, you're less likely to bite them. And if your hands look beautiful, you're less likely to want to cover them up (as most nail-biters tend to do).

## 706 HARD AS NAILS

For weak or brittle nails, apply a nail strengthener every day for a week, then remove and leave the nails to rest for a few days before repeating for another week, if necessary. Make sure you file the nails into a square shape rather than an oval, which will avoid weakening the sides and causing splits and tears.

## 707 CARE FOR CUTICLES

Massage a cuticle oil or cream into the base of the nails at least once a day to prevent dryness, scarring and hangnails. If cuticles are damaged and painful, gently apply a moisturizer twice daily until they heal.

## 708 BUFF AWAY RIDGES

Ridges on the nail are mostly down to genetics but although you can't change them, you can smooth the ridged nail surface with a buffer and buffing cream.

## 709 CHECK YOUR IRON LEVELS

If you've recently developed ridges on your nails, which you haven't suffered before, it could be a sign of anaemia and you should consult your doctor. On the other hand, it might be the result of an over-zealous manicurist, so don't panic just yet!

## 710 TWINKLE THOSE TOES

Pale, subtle varnishes are wasted on summer toenails – open-toed sandals cry out for bright colours, such as shocking pink, or sparkly and metallic hues.

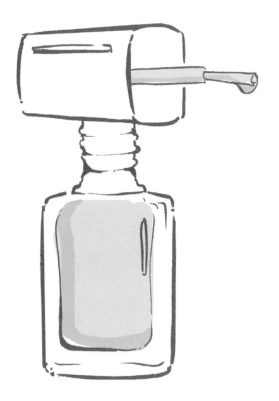

## 711 FILE WITHOUT FRICTION

When filing nails, work in one direction from the outside edge toward the centre, rather than sawing back and forth, as too much friction can cause splits and tears. Angle the file slightly so you are filing away more from underneath the nail than on top. Avoid metal emery boards, which can be too harsh for nail ends.

## 712 LET SPOTS GROW OUT

White spots on nails are usually the result of trauma to the nail or nail bed. Give the spots time to grow out and make an effort to be gentle when manicuring your nails – prodding beneath the cuticles, where new growth is generated, can cause white spots and damaged nails.

## 713 BACK TO BASES

If you have yellow nails, it could be because you haven't used a base coat underneath your regular nail colour. Yellow patches or streaks that don't go away could be due to fungal infections that might need treatment.

## 714 LIGHTEN UP WITH LEMON

Lighten discoloured nails with a whitening scrub containing a mild abrasive or with a remover containing lemon juice to bleach out colour. Ask your local manicurist or chemist for product recommendations.

## 715 FAKE IT 'TIL YOU MAKE IT

A sure fire way to stop biting your nails is to invest in a pair of falsies. Your teeth won't like the feel of the acrylic nail fibres and it will help you kick the habit. Plus, your nails will look great!

## 716 SEAL IN DRY NAILS

To protect nails from drying, use a waterproof varnish that seals moisture in the nail and repels water and dirt. A waxy lip balm or nail oil can also be quite effective at moisturizing nails overnight.

## 717 CHILL OUT

Nail varnish will stay fresher for longer if it's kept in the refrigerator, which will help prevent it separating and clogging due to heat and light damage.

## 718 LET YOUR NAILS BREATHE

Leave nails unpainted for at least a few days a month to help them breathe. This will reduce yellowing and staining from polish on the nail and give it a chance to recover health and glow.

## 719 CUT AWAY HANGNAILS

Picking and biting your nails, exposing them to detergents and chemicals, and a lack of general nail maintenance are all causes of hangnails. Use a pair of sharp cuticle scissors to remove existing hangnails, cutting close to the skin.

## 720 ELEGANCE AT YOUR FINGERTIPS

If your nails are on the short side, give an illusion of length by leaving a narrow strip of bare nail on each side when applying varnish. This will instantly narrow your nails.

## 721 WHITEN YOUR TIPS

If you haven't got time to paint your nails, fill in the underside of nail tips with a white nail pencil, which can give a naturally glamorous boost to unpainted nails.

## 722 CLING ON

Wait at least 45 minutes after painting your toenails before putting on closed-toe shoes, but if you absolutely must go out, wrap your toes in plastic wrap before slipping on shoes to avoid smudges.

## 723 BE A SQUARE

Clip and file toenails squarely in line with the ends of the toes so that the growth does not push into the surrounding tissue, which can be ugly and painful.

## 724 PAINT LIKE A PRO

To help nails look long and strong, start the polish in a curve in line with, and just above, the cuticle. Avoid getting polish on the cuticle, which shortens nails. If you slip, use a cotton bud to remove excess polish.

## 725 ZAP FLECKS WITH ZINC

White flecks in the nails are caused by injury or, in some cases, a deficiency of zinc. Supplement your diet with eggs, shellfish, chickpeas and lentils, all good sources of dietary zinc.

## 726 OPT FOR ACETONE-FREE

To remove nail varnish, choose an acetone-free remover, which will lift off the colour without drying or damaging the nail surface. Acetone removers can strip nails of natural oils, making them dry and dull.

## 727 DON'T CUT CUTICLES

Instead of cutting cuticles, which can cause them to become hard and scarred, soak hands and push them back with a flannel or towel, then apply a cuticle oil or cream to keep them soft.

## 728 SMOOTH OUT NAILS

To avoid ridges and irregularities in the nail surface, apply a base coat before nail varnish or colour, which will also provide a protective layer and prevent staining.

## 729 THINK THIN

Polish that peels from the edge of the nail is usually due to the layers having been too thickly applied. Rather than one or two thick coats, try larger numbers of thinner coats instead.

## 730 COLOUR THAT LASTS

Colour wears off the tips of polished nails first. To make your manicure last longer, take the colour over the edge of the nail to underneath – the added polish will protect against chipping.

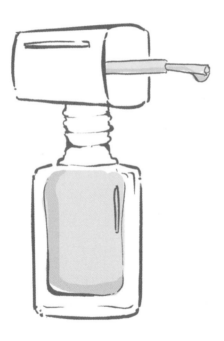

# salon secrets

## 731 TIP YOUR THERAPIST

If you liked the therapy and want the same person next time, give them a ten per cent tip as you leave to show your appreciation. They'll find space in their schedule for you if you want another appointment!

## 732 BRAVE MICRODERMABRASION

This skin-booster uses aluminium oxide particles to slough off the outermost layers, leaving complexions brighter and evening out tone and colour. There are home-based alternatives, but professional is best to reduce redness and irritation post-treatment.

## 733 LASER YOUR VEINS

The treatment works by using lasers to create heat in the veins, which damages the lining of the blood vessel and causes the walls of the vessel to stick together and seal themselves off. The vein is gradually absorbed by the body and disappear.

## 734 DIP INTO THE DEAD SEA

You can buy these products for use at home, but the more powerful ingredients are reserved for salon formulations. The treatments use the mineral-rich mud from the Dead Sea to detoxify and revitalize skin.

## 735 HARVEST YOUR OWN CELLS

An alternative to Botox that uses your own skin cells, Isolagen treatments takes a tiny skin cell sample from behind your ear. The cells are grown in a lab and re-injected into frown lines, crow's feet and wrinkly hands. They are used medically to heal scarring from burns. You are using your own, younger skin cells, preserved cyrogenically, to rejuvenate your skin as you Four or more treatments are needed to see the benefits.

## 736 BEAT LINES WITH BOTOX

Botox can be administered in a lunch break and it's considered fairly safe, if done by experts, with few complications. The botulinum toxin is injected into the forehead and crow's feet to paralyze muscles. Results last about three months.

## 737 PEEL AWAY PROBLEMS

Facial chemical peels should always be performed by a trained therapist or dermatologist, as the concentrations of skin-clearing chemicals are higher than in home-based treatments, which means they penetrate more deeply and have more radical results.

## 738 DON'T BE FAZED BY LASERS

Lasers are now being used in salons to resurface, smooth and lighten skin and to even out pigmentation, age marks and acne scars. Because lasers can inflict damage, you should always visit a professional to have them administered.

## 739 BE ALERT TO ALLERGIES

If you're allergic to shellfish, tell your beauty therapist before beginning any treatments. Many face products and wraps contain ground shells or marine products, which could cause an allergic reaction, such as redness or swelling. As a matter of course, always warn the therapist about all allergies, sensitivities and medical conditions.

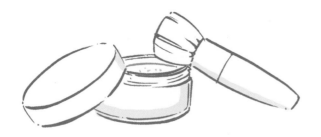

## 741 SEE IMPROVEMENTS WITH CACI

CACI facials tighten and tone skin by introducing an electrical current to points on your face. Sagging muscles and skin tissues are stimulated and the benefits can be seen after several treatments.

## 740 QUICK-TIME MAKEOVERS

If you are time-poor and need a quick makeover for a special event, book an express treatment. Many hair and beauty salons offer a cut and colour combined with body treatments, such as manicures, massages and brow shaping.

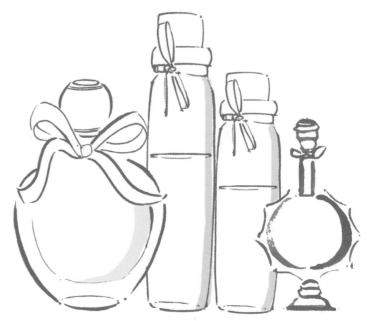

## 742 TIGHT AND FIRM

Thermage and Thermacool treatments work by heating the underlying tissues of the skin, causing the collagen to contract so your skin firms and wrinkles smooth out.

## 743 CACI YOUR ASSETS

CACI technology isn't just used for the face – it can also be used to create a nonsurgical 'bust lift' by targeting sagging skin on the chest and firming the bust.

## 744 SMOOTH SPOTS WITH SMOOTHBEAM

A good salon choice for spotty or greasy skins, smoothbeam lasers are used to target oil glands, which slows down oil production, helping prevent spots and blackheads, and to stimulate collagen production, which can tighten pores.

## 745 BE A BOLD BRAZILIAN

A Brazilian bikini wax, which leaves just a tiny 'landing strip' of hair on the delicate pubic area, is best left to professionals because they have the skills to prevent bruising and to minimize pain.

## 746 FILL IT WITH FILLERS

To fill out acne scars, frown lines and wrinkles, dermal fillers are popular for the areas Botox doesn't reach – such as the laugh lines and for pumping up thin lips. Choose a biodegradable hyaluronic acid-based filler rather than a permanent one – the results last less time but there is less chance of unsightly lumps and movement.

## 747 MASSAGE AWAY PUFFINESS

A great instant pick-me-up if you are suffering from puffy or problem skin is a manual lymphatic drainage (MLD) massage, which boosts circulation, detoxifies and reduces fluid build-up. It is used to improve cellulite and stretch marks, too.

## 748 BOOST YOUR OXYGEN

A fabulous salon treatment loved by models is a facial designed to boost the oxygen levels in your skin by pumping oxygen onto the face via a metal tube from a tank. It leaves a genuine (if short-lived) glow and skin feels rejuvenated. To stimulate the effect, try oxygen creams.

## 748 ASK FOR A JEWEL

Some skin conditions can respond to electronic gem therapy, which involves passing light rays through gemstones. For eczema sufferers, emeralds and sapphires are used to zap problem areas.

## 750 LIGHT UP YOUR LIFE

New salon treatments that involve an application of yellow light to reduce the bacterial count in skin can reduce acne by up to half after just one treatment. Called Light Therapy, it's a miracle for problem skin.

## 751 THERMO-TARGET THREAD VEINS

Thermo-coagulation is a vein-removal technique based on a high-frequency wave producing a thermal lesion that reduces the vein. A very fine needle is inserted into the vein and it disappears instantaneously.

## 752 PIECE OF THE ACTION

GABA is a surface-applied ingredient that has been used pharmaceutically to freeze muscles, mimicking the effects of Botox without an invasive injection.

## 753 A NICE LITTLE LEARNER

If you're stuck in a rut, book a lesson with a top make-up artist. They can teach you professional tricks and introduce you to new colours and products. Boutiques and salons also have staff on hand for lessons but the smaller ones tend to be less hectic and more individualistic than those at big department stores.

## 754 SHARE IN A FLOTATION

Your bath is just too small for a flotation experience so a salon visit is a must. Excellent for toning and relaxing, flotation entails floating in darkness in a special tank. The treatment helps your body and mind relax in peace and harmony.

## 755 HANDLE HYLAFORM WITH CARE

Dermal injections involve plumping up facial lines and wrinkles by injecting small amounts of the filler into them. Hylaform uses hyaluronic acid, from rooster combs, as its key compound, which could cause allergic reactions. Non-animal derived hyaluronic is used in Restylane and Perlane.

## 756 HOT SUGAR BODY POLISH

Don't try this at home, unless you're prepared to caramelize yourself. A hot sugar solution is applied to the skin and all-over massage is used to stimulate circulation and make the skin glow.

## 757 OPT FOR SCLEROTHERAPY

Sclerotherapy removes thread veins from the legs by injecting a special solution into the vein via an ultra-fine needle. The sides of the vein stick together and the vein eventually fades away. The smaller the vein, the easier it is to treat. It may also remedy such symptoms as aching, burning, swelling and cramps.

## 758 PULSE AWAY PIGMENT

Pulsed light technology is an alternative to lasers. With this salon treatment, pulses of intense, concentrated light are directed onto the skin and absorbed by the melanin in pigmented lesions, such as age, sun and liver spots, which evens out pigmentation. The technique is also used for hair removal and blemishes.

# smooth & firm

## 759 BALANCE OUT BREASTS

If you have uneven breasts, don't worry – most women do. Try an enhanced bra with the enhancement taken out of the cup that holds the larger breast, or use one of those 'chicken fillet' external implants.

## 760 LOOK LEAN BY GOING GREEN

Did you know that green tea can help you lose weight by stimulating your basal metabolic rate to help you burn calories more easily? Two cups a day is ample.

## 761 GIVE YOURSELF THE BRUSH-OFF

Improving skin circulation – by body brushing, scrubbing and massage – will even out skin tone and boost oxygenation of the cells, leading to fresher, smoother, glowing skin all year round.

## 762 BE COOL

Hot showers can sting skin and cause moisture loss. Instead, finish off hot days with a lukewarm or tepid shower blast.

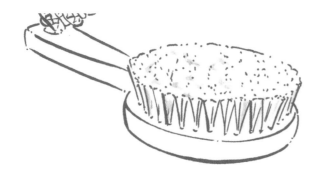

## 763 BRUSH AWAY BLEMISHES

Dry body brushing kickstarts the circulation and aids the elimination of toxins, which prevents skin looking puffy and helps you avoid blemishes, spots and dry patches, especially those white bumps that appear on the arms and legs that are a sign of congested skin.

## 764 STAND UP STRAIGHT

Improve your bust line simply by standing up straighter. Improved posture will naturally lift the ribcage and enable the breasts to sit more upright on the chest. Imagine a golden string through your spine, pulling your head upwards.

## 765 FIRM WITH A GEL

The delicate skin on the neck and upper chest is a target for sun damage and ages fast. In fact, you may notice the neck lines and crevices before you notice them on your face. The best formulas for this area are gel- or serum-based and not only deliver a sunscreen and anti-ageing moisturizer, but fade age spots and firm loose skin, albeit temporarily.

## 766 BUST TONERS

Toners formulated for tightening the bust area have an instant but temporary effect, though the ingredients they deliver have longterm benefits for skin health. Though there is no nonsurgical route to a bust lift, these treatments can assist in cell metabolism and strengthen and renew the skin to leave the texture refined. Massage in gently, avoiding the nipples.

## 767 TAKE UP ARMS

Regular massage will help prevent rough skin and pimples on the arms. Massage in almond or olive oil to boost circulation and concentrate on the back of arms, where fat deposits can cause uneven skin.

## 768 ALL FOR ALMOND OIL

Use sweet almond oil after a bath or shower to coat the body in the vitamin A-rich oil, which the skin will absorb where it needs it. An excellent, penetrating emollient, it is useful for all skin types and relieves itching and irritation. Concentrate particularly on dry areas and, if possible, leave on overnight.

## 769 GRAB A GRAPEFRUIT

Grapefruit is an excellent choice for a healthy fruit that will make you look good. It is a natural diuretic, which prevents bloating and water retention, and helps you stay slim. Choose it as a healthy starter or a mid-afternoon snack. Many beauty products contain grapefruit purely for its reinvigorating scent.

## 770 GET SLICK WITH LOTION

To give yourself an extra watery boost and lock in extra moisture, slather on moisturizing creams directly after a bath or shower while your skin is still damp. Body creams and lotions that contain gentle chemical exfoliators, including glycolic acid and salicylic acid can help even out skin tone, while 'contouring' or 'lifting' creams will improve skin texture.

## 771 BEAT THE BLOAT

Stock up your diet with natural diuretics. Watercress, watermelon, fennel and peppermint tea can all stop your body bloating and retaining water, which can make eyes and cheeks look puffy – as well as your tummy – and add pounds.

## 772 MASSAGE AS YOU MOISTURIZE

When you apply a body oil or lotion, do so using massage techniques: use sweeping, upward motions towards your heart to give your lymphatic drainage a boost. Taking time to really work the oil into your skin will help it penetrate and imbue a lustrous glow.

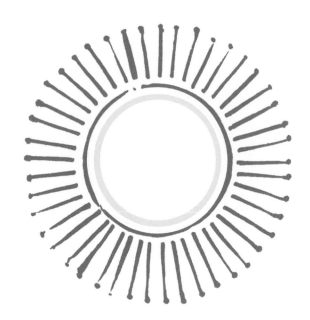

# sun worship

## 773 THROW ON THE TOWEL

If you burn the skin on your face, place a damp, cold flannel over the burnt area for ten minutes to take away redness and swelling. Avoid alcohol, smoke and further sun until the redness fades, and use aftersun moisturizer twice a day.

## 774 HEAD FOR A SCREEN TEST

Don't be tempted to use intensive moisturizers or conditioners in your hair in the hope that they'll keep your locks protected in the sun – the sun burns them up, which can make hair even drier. Instead, use a hair-specific sunscreen for ultimate protection.

## 775 BE A SHADY LADY

Take care of the delicate skin around the eyes with a pair of polarized sunglasses. Wraparound styles that fully cover the whole eye area and the sides of the face are best, as they protect the skin prone to crows' feet and fine under-eye lines.

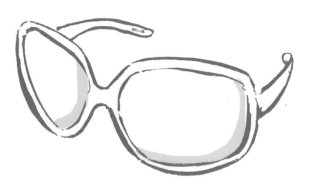

## 776 CHUCK IT AFTER A YEAR

Sunscreen loses its protective power after a yea. When the summer's over, throw away those sunscreens so you're not tempted to re-use them next year.

## 777 KEEP CREAM COOL

Sun cream is more effective when it's kept cool, so make sure you leave it in the shade if you're on the beach, or the sun's heat could denature the active ingredients and make it less effective.

## 778 DON'T GO FOR THE BURN

Not only is burnt skin dangerous, it will peel faster, leaving you with pink patches and a dry, flaky surface. Use suntan lotions and creams with added moisturizers and pace yourself with sun exposure for a smooth, even tan.

## 779 BE A CITY SLICKER

Skin isn't only exposed to the sun on the beach in summer – in town choose a tinted moisturizer with built-in sunscreen to give you a healthy glow without the damage.

## 780 LET'S GET THIS CLEAR

For beautiful beach skin, go for the model's choice – a clear or yellow-tinged sunscreen with a high factor instead of the white lotions that make your skin appear pale and pasty. These varieties will give your skin a golden appearance while delivering high protection at the same time. Sprays are best for even coverage.

## 781 GET PHYSICAL

If you have sensitive skin, allergies or acne, opt for a physical sunscreen that contains mineral ingredients to block out the rays rather than a chemical-based version containing parabens, which have been shown to increase skin sensitivity.

## 782 DO THE DOSE RIGHT

For a sunscreen to live up to its SPF rating, 2 mg should be applied for every square centimetre (½ inch) of exposed skin, which means on average you should be using 100 mg for every four whole-body applications. Most people don't use anything like enough.

### 783 DON'T BE HASTY

When you moisturize before applying a sunscreen, make sure you leave 15–30 minutes for the moisturizer to soak into the skin first. This will ensure that the sunblock works correctly.

### 784 MAKE UP IF YOU MUST

If you really can't brave the beach without make-up, apply waterproof cosmetics first and then pat sunblock over the top to ensure even protection and to prevent make-up from sliding down your face. Avoid full foundation, opting instead for a touch of concealer. Consider having your eyelashes and brows (if pale) tinted to keep your features from looking faded in the sun.

### 785 KEEP HAIR SMOOTH

UV rays, chlorine and salt can damage and dry hair, so protect hair as well as skin in the sun using a sunscreen spray, mask or cream specially formulated for the hair. These products will lock moisture in and reduce colour fade.

### 786 START EARLY IF YOU'RE ACTIVE

If you're going to be active on sunny days and are worried about sweating off your sunscreen, make sure you apply it at least half an hour before you expose yourself to make sure your skin has absorbed it.

### 787 JOIN THE BAND

Worried about sun damage? Invest in a UV wristband, a disposable band you wear on your wrist that measures sun exposure and turns colour when you've had enough.

### 788 BE AN A-LIST STAR

It's not just your suncream's UVB-protective SPF rating that counts – make sure your cream's got a UVA-blocking star rating as well. It goes from one to five, with five being the strongest.

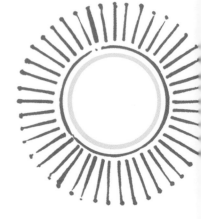

## 789 TAN WITH TANGERINES

Antioxidant vitamins A, C and E – found in red, yellow and orange fruit and vegetables – can help limit damage to skin from the sun's rays by mopping up damaging free radicals in the body.

## 780 PROTECT YOUR FACE

The skin on your face and neck is among the thinnest and most sensitive on your body. To prevent damage from the sun's rays, cover up with a wide-brimmed hat, especially in the danger hours from 11 am to 3 pm. This will also protect your hair from looking sun-frazzled.

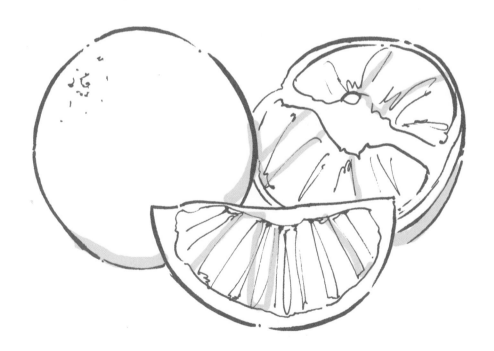

## 781 PUCKER UP

Don't forget lips need sun protection too – the skin on them is thinner than anywhere else on your face, and overexposure to the sun and elements can leave them dry and coarse. Use a sunscreen specially formulated for the lips with a minimum of SPF 15.

## 782 COOL DOWN SUMMER BURN

Chlorine, sun and high temperatures can make the skin on your legs more prone to post-shave stinging and rashes. Use a lotion with aloe vera to soothe – studies have shown that aloe vera improves the skin's ability to hydrate itself and that it speeds healing. Store the lotion in the fridge for 20 minutes before application for a soothing treat that will really cool skin.

## 783 WITCH WAY TO STOP THE ITCH?

Ease sunburnt areas and prevent itching, soreness and further damage with a homemade body lotion. Mix 120 ml (4 fl oz) of witch hazel with 60 ml (2 fl oz) each of aloe vera gel, baby oil and high-factor sunscreen.

# sunless tanning

## 784 DO YOUR PREP

Self-tanners contain a chemical called DHA (dihydroxyacetone), a colourless sugar that stains the uppermost layer of skin, so it's better to get the application right in the first place than try to correct mistakes. Try the 3-step rule: exfoliate, moisturize, apply.

## 785 RUB AWAY STREAKS

For overdone or streaky self-tan, exfoliate the area with a creamy scrub to slough away dead skin cells and reduce blotches.

## 786 HANDS OFF THE TAN!

Prevent tell-tale orange palms by applying a tiny amount of silicone-based 'frizz-control' hair product to your palms, which blocks the pigment from absorbing into your skin.

## 787 DRY SKIN MAY GO DARK

Dry skin around knees, elbows and ankles picks up self-tan colour more, leading to dark patches. Instead of applying tan neat, mix it with moisturizer for these areas.

## 798 FAKE IT FLAWLESSLY

When you're choosing a fake tan lotion, look for one that contains erythrulose, a unique DHA enhancer. The combination of DHA and erythrulose helps ensure a more even, streakless, longlasting tan without increasing dryness.

## 799 STOP THE FADE

Keep your fake tan looking great all week by avoiding moisturizers that contain any of the following: Retin-A, AHAs, BHAs or glycolic acids. These ingredients will slough off the dead cells in the top layer of the skin and make your tan fade faster.

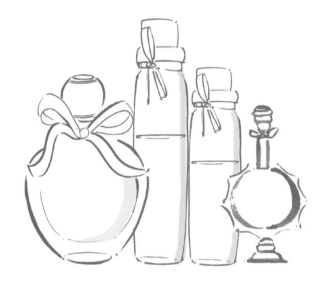

## 800 EXFOLIATE DAILY

Prepare your skin for self-tanning by exfoliating daily for the three or four days before you apply it and using moisturizer liberally following exfoliation to build up smoothness and hydration in the skin and prevent uneven streaks.

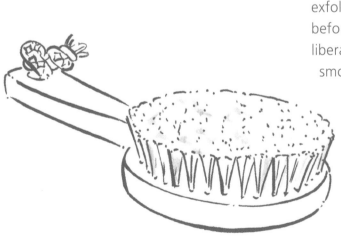

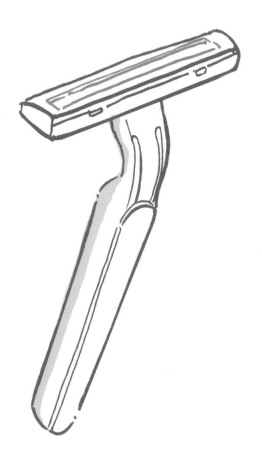

### 801 FAKE TANNING FOR BLONDES

After applying fake tan to the face, sweep a tissue around the hairline and over the brows to avoid colouring light hair. Don't forget to scrub the nails and palms of the hands afterwards, too.

### 802 HAVE A CLOSE SHAVE

Shaving not only removes hairs, it also serves to exfoliate the skin by stretching off the top layer, so it's a great choice the day before you apply self-tan. But avoid shaving for a day or two afterwards as it could weaken the tan.

### 803 MOISTURIZE MODERATELY

Too much moisturizer is one of the biggest fake tan mistakes – it creates a barrier between the skin and the tan, making the tanning dye less effective and more prone to slipping and streaks. Wait until the body cream has soaked in before applying fake tan.

### 804 BUILD UP TO SUCCESS

Perfect the no-streaks, natural-looking tan with a little patience! Instead of slathering it all on at once, apply a light layer of self-tan at a time and build up the colour with a second application a few days later.

### 805 HIDE THE TIDE MARK

If tan lines caused by bikinis, tops, shorts and socks are blighting your quest for the all-over tan, smooth out marks by applying small amounts of fake tan (mixed with moisturizer at first so you don't go too dark) to give yourself an even-looking tan. Simply reapply as the tan fades.

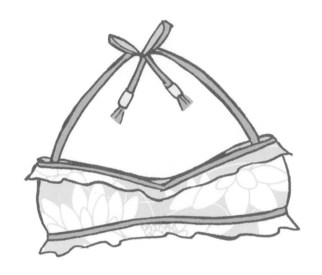

### 806 SPRAY-ON SUN

Modern airbrush spray-tanning booths will give you an all-over aloe-based DHA tan without your body ever seeing the sun. One session will last about a week and you can choose from a range of shades. A good idea to ease yourself from a tan into a wintry pallor is to invest in a series of sessions – a once-a-week session will keep your tan going for months to come.

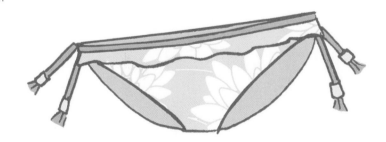

## inner beauty

### 807 GET FRESH BREATH

When you don't have a toothbrush handy, or when you've indulged in a lunchtime meal of garlic, eat a pot of natural live yogurt. The yogurt will neutralize nasty smells and leave your breath super-fresh.

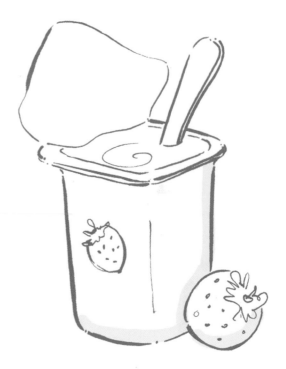

## 808 COUNT YOUR UNITS

Alcohol causes changes in the body's circulation system, which can lead to broken veins on cheeks and nose. Keep your intake down to a maximum of 14 units a week and try to have at least one completely dry day.

## 809 POLISH WITH PORRIDGE

For a morning glow, breakfast on porridge with skimmed milk, topped with flaxseeds and blueberries and a glass of orange juice, – all the best ingredients for healthy skin.

## 810 SCOFF FRUIT FOR HEALTHY SKIN

Fruit is essential for healthy skin, not only because of all the vitamins and minerals, but also because it contains high levels of water, which also serve to keep skin hydrated. Pimples or congested skin in the forehead area is often a sign of constipation or blockage in the lymphatic systems, which can be relieved by eating plenty of fruit and vegetables.

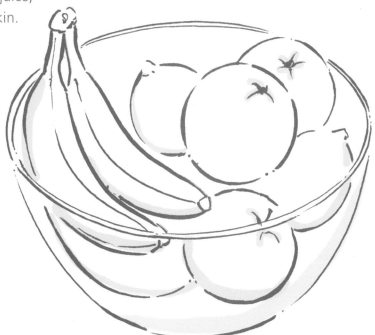

## 811 BREATHE YOURSELF BEAUTIFUL

Breathing properly is key to beautiful skin, hair and nails because it encourages higher levels of oxygen into your system. To ensure you're breathing deeply, place your hands on your belly and feel it expand as you take an in-breath, and deflate as you breathe out naturally. To start each day relaxed and calm, take a few minutes each morning to close your eyes and concentrate on your breathing.

## 812 ROAR LIKE A LION

Use the yoga position called the Lion to keep your face and neck vibrant and toned. Take a deep breath and, as you breathe out, open your mouth as wide as possible and stick out your tongue. Move your eyes (but not your head) to look at the ceiling, without straining them, and hold for a count of eight.

## 813 MIX UP A BEAUTY SNACK

Fix yourself a mini-meal of low-fat muesli mixed with ground flaxseeds and dried fruit, topped with plain yogurt. For another beauty-boosting snack drink tomato juice with a splash of lemon.

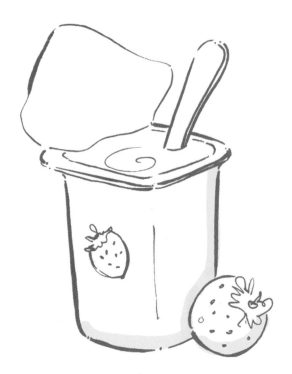

### 814 GO FOR GRAPEFRUIT

Eat well for gorgeous-looking skin, by fixing yourself a lunch of grilled shrimp salad with grapefruit and watercress. These ingredients contain high levels of zinc and antioxidants to boost skin healing. Top it with parsley, which is rich in vitamin A, chlorophyll, vitamin B12, folic acid, vitamin C and iron – all good for skin health.

### 815 BOOST YOUR CONFIDENCE

Believing in your own good looks will make others believe in them, too. Presenting a positive mental attitude and self assurance will help you exude attractiveness. If you don't always feel it, try pretending to be confident and good-looking – it can make a big difference to how others perceive you.

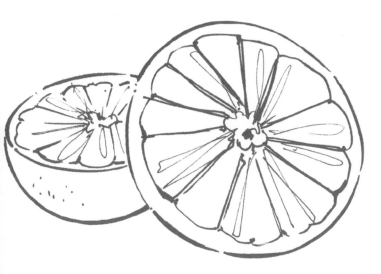

# natural remedies

### 816 PASS THE PARSLEY JUICE

Natural parsley juice (or parsley infusion) mixed with equal amounts of lemon juice, orange juice and redcurrant juice can be applied under your favourite face cream to keep freckles and other pigment spots less visible – the vitamin C in parsley regulates melanin production and evens skin tone. An infusion of fresh parsley can also be used to cleanse the skin to help clear acne.

## 817 HYDRATE WITH FRUITS AND NUTS

For extra-dry, scaly or flaky skin, look for products that contain sweet almond oil, apricot and berries like blackberry, all of which pack a super-hydrating punch and will help regenerate tissues without blocking pores.

## 818 PUT ON THE PARSLEY

Parsley is a great natural remedy for spots and blackheads because of its circulation-boosting properties. Grind the fresh herbs into a pulp and use as a face mask. Leave on for 10–15 minutes before rinsing off.

## 819 THE THYME IS RIGHT

Thyme contains deep-cleansing elements that remove dirt and debris in the skin. It also kills bacteria, which can cause acne, so an infusion is perfect for cleansing problem skin.

## 820 EMULATE AN EMU FOR SHINY HAIR

Emu oil is rich in omega-3 oils, which make your hair shiny and healthy. It is available in supplement or oil form, which you apply as a mask or conditioner.

## 821 CLEANSE WITH CARING OILS

Rather than invest in expensive creams, try a simple, natural cleanser, particularly good for mature skins. Apply a light film of almond or wheatgerm oil over your face, leave for a minute then remove with a warm damp cloth or natural sponge.

## 822 HOME IN ON HOMEOPATHY

Homeopathic urtica tablets are derived from the stinging nettle, which not only has calming properties but also contains antihistamines, which naturally reduce the effects of allergic reactions.

## 823 CUT SUGAR FOR CLEAR SKIN

Sugar, refined carbohydrates and saturated fats can contribute to blemishes. If you think your diet is to blame, try a gentle detox programme to purify your system.

## 824 ALMOND EYES

Almond oil is a super all-round moisturizer. Use it on your lips and around your mouth, as a hand moisturizer or as a gentle eye make-up remover to smooth away wrinkles.

## 825 END ITCHING WITH ALOE

For those suffering extreme dryness or eczema, creams containing high levels of lavender and aloe vera can stop the itching. These ingredients have fast-acting, skin-soothing properties.

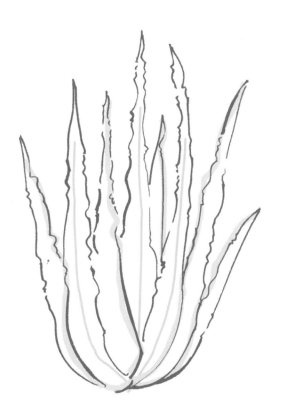

## 826 CURE SPOTS WITH FENUGREEK

Fenugreek leaves infused in a small amount of water and made into a paste can be used to target pimples, blackheads and dryness if applied and left overnight. Wash off with warm water in the morning.

## 827 COME TO THE OIL

Essential oils are relaxing, detoxifying and nourishing. They are absorbed very easily and won't leave your face shiny. Rose oil is particularly noted for its soothing properties and restores suppleness to mature skins – blend a few drops with patchouli and geranium oils in a carrier oil and apply a small amount nightly.

## 828 JOJOBA FOR HAIR DRYNESS

Jojoba oil is waxy and rich in antioxidants; it will condition and nourish the hair shaft, leaving hair moisturized, smooth and sleek. Leave on overnight for a deep treatment, shampooing it out in the morning, or look for conditioner that contains it. Although plant-derived, jojoba is closer in makeup to sebum than to traditional vegetable oils.

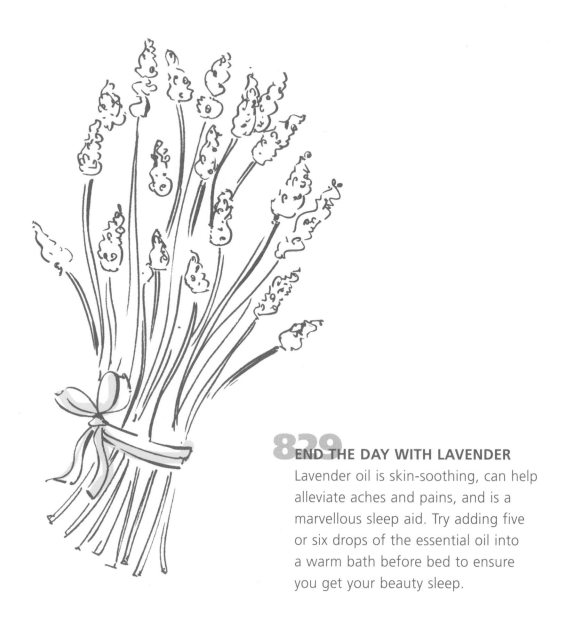

## 829 END THE DAY WITH LAVENDER

Lavender oil is skin-soothing, can help alleviate aches and pains, and is a marvellous sleep aid. Try adding five or six drops of the essential oil into a warm bath before bed to ensure you get your beauty sleep.

## 830 BOOST SKIN HEALTH WITH APRICOTS

Apricots are a rich source of betacarotene, folic acid and iron, all of which boost skin health and help combat damaging free radicals and toxins from the environment and additives in food and cosmetics. The vitamin A helps keep skin soft and supple, and repairs skin cells and tissues.

## 831 RITES OF MASSAGE

Massage can help uneven skin tone by boosting circulation and encouraging the migration of pigment cells under the skin, which evens out patchiness. It is especially good for circulation danger spots like the chin, jaw and upper arms.

## 832 PRESS AWAY PROBLEMS

In acupuncture, the area above your kneecap (measure the length of your kneecap and move exactly this distance above it and 2.5 cm (1in) towards your inner thigh) is linked to skin problems. Press on each leg at the spot for at least a minute to reduce itching and inflammation of the skin.

## 833 GET EVEN WITH PRIMROSE

Many natural cosmetics include evening primrose oil as one of their key components. The oil has a high concentration of omega-3 oils and gamma-linolenic acid (GLA) that have been shown to help prevent and ease symptoms of psoriasis, eczema and other skin conditions. It also helps maintain the skin's water barrier. The essential fatty acids keep nails healthy and prevent cracks, and nourish the scalp and hair.

## 834 SOOTHE SKIN WITH ALMONDS

Almond oil and ground almonds mixed with water are excellent ways to treat problem skin because of their gentle soothing properties, calming irritated nerve endings and reducing spotty outbreaks.

## 835 SEARCH FOR WHITE BIRCH

White birch contains powerful lightening ingredients in the bark, which have been shown to work equally well on the skin. Used regularly, white birch can reduce areas of pigmentation and help make skin appear more even in colour.

## 836 CAST YOUR OATS

Rather than spend money on expensive exfoliants, grab some oats from your kitchen cupboard. Crush them into a paste with some water and rub lightly over the face and neck for natural exfoliation and a healthy glow. Do not use on sensitive skins.

## 837 BE AN OMEGA-3 BEAUTY

Omega-3 oils, found in high levels in oily fish like mackerel, sardines and salmon, can benefit skin by reducing inflammation and helping the elimination of toxins.

## 838 COOL AS A CUCUMBER

Cucumber juice is good for blemishes because it refreshes and keeps skin hydrated without drying. It has mild astringent qualities that can help reduce redness and swelling, which makes spots look worse.

## 839 OVERCOME ITCHING WITH OATS

Oats contain natural anti-inflammatory properties which can help reduce skin flare-ups. For a simple home remedy, add a few cups of oats to a warm bath and wallow for 15 minutes to calm problem skin.

## 840 ORGANIZE AN ORGANIC DIET

Some scientists think that sensitive skin could be made worse by too many additives, colourings and preservatives in foods. If your skin is red or inflamed, try eating lots of natural, organic foods.

## 841 SEED THE BENEFITS

Pumpkin, sesame and sunflower seeds are packed with skin-rejuvenating elements like essential fats, vitamins and minerals. Include them in your diet at least three or four times a week for best results.

## 842 EASE ECZEMA WITH LINOLEIC ACID

Linoleic acid, found in many supplements and most nuts and seeds, is a powerful omega-6 oil, which helps eczema sufferers more than olive or fish oils.

## 843 CHOOSE THE GREY HAIR HERB

Fo ti, also known as the 'grey hair herb', is claimed to darken and reduce the appearance of grey hair with regular use. It is available as a supplement, oil or ingredient in hair products.

## 844 SLEEP WELL WITH SANDALWOOD

As well as being an excellent moisturizer, a few drops of sandalwood oil in your bath can help decrease tension and relieve insomnia. Traditionally, it is also a natural antidepressant.

## 845 SALT OF THE EARTH

Salt baths encourage gentle detoxification of your whole body, and are particularly good for problem skin and fluid retention. Taken at the end of the day, they can also reduce tension and promote a good night's sleep.

## 846 IN THE PINK WITH ZINC

Zinc, which can be taken as a supplement or found in foods such as red meat, shellfish, sunflower seeds and peanuts, can help you keep skin clear and spot-free by boosting circulation and toxin removal.

## 847 TEA TREE WORKS A TREAT

Lavender and tea tree oil, as well as witch hazel, have natural antiseptic properties that can help prevent spots and bites becoming infected. Manuka honey is also a natural antiseptic, though it's a lot stickier!

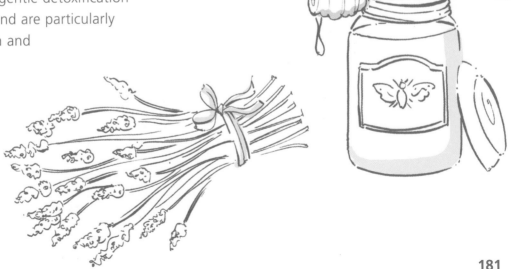

## 848 SIP CAMOMILE FOR BEAUTIFUL EYES

Drinking camomile tea before bed is a good way to reduce under-eye bags, both by helping you get your beauty sleep and by reducing facial tension, which can cause dark circles to form.

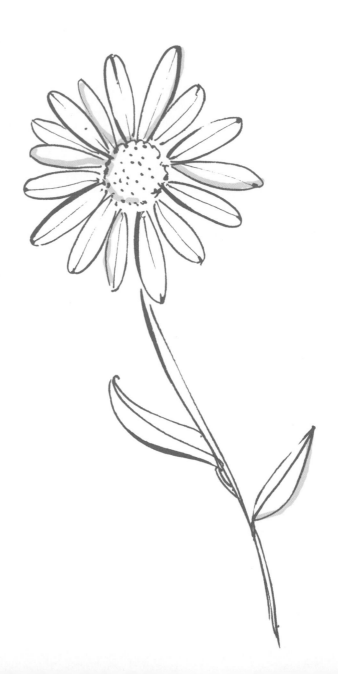

# supplements

## 849 AFA FOR HEALTHY HAIR

The supplement AFA (aphanizomenon flos-aquae) is a blue-green algae that contains all eight essential amino acids. It gives shine to hair, stimulates nail health, increases mental and physical alertness, promotes healthy intestinal flora and provides stable blood sugar levels.

## 850 GET THE MSM MESSAGE

MSM (methylsulfonylmethane) is a naturally occurring nutrient found in protein-rich eggs, meat and fish. It is often called nature's beauty mineral, as it promotes a clear complexion, glossy hair and fast and effective recovery from injury, including scar healing.

## 851 B FREE OF LIVER SPOTS

A supplement high in B vitamins is thought to help clear up liver spots on face and hands, which can be unsightly. You can also find B vitamins in meat, fortified cereals and yeast extract.

## 852 BE A GREENIE

Daily sipping of green tea could help you stay looking slimmer and fitter by reducing cellulite through its effects on the body's metabolic rate. It does contain caffeine, though, so don't overdo it.

## 853 WHEATGRASS

Loaded with vitamins, minerals, amino acids and enzymes, wheatgrass juice can be taken as a drink, applied to the skin or taken as a supplement. As a toner it will fade blemishes and sunspots, stimulate the growth of healthy new skin, and

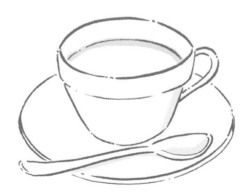

## 854 SUPPLEMENTS CAN SALVE PSORIASIS

Psoriasis, which leaves dry, scaly patches on the skin, can be relieved by taking daily supplements of evening primrose oil, vitamin E and/or cod liver oil to help the skin replenish its moisture levels.

## 855 BE A COD LIVER LOVER

Cod liver oil has long been used by women to maintain beautiful skins. It helps to regulate the natural oils in the skin, preventing dryness without making it feel greasy or causing spots and blemishes.

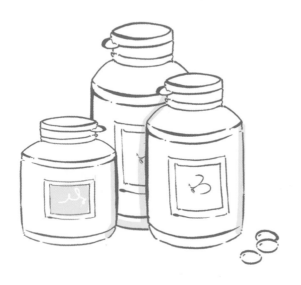

## 856 ZAP SPOTS WITH SPIRULINA

Spirulina is a blue-green algae that contains high levels of amino acids and antioxidants, probiotics and phytonutrients – which can be passed on to our bodies to promote healthy skin and hair. Taken as supplements or used as a mask, it is thought to work against blemish formation.

## 857 HORSE AROUND

Horse chestnut is an age-old remedy for treating varicose veins, haemorrhoids and other problems linked with poor circulation. Take it in tablet form to boost and tone of your circulatory system.

## 858 BEAT SPOTS WITH EVENING PRIMROSE

Evening primrose oil, taken as daily capsules, has been shown to help skin stay supple and spot-free as well as to beat the signs of PMS, which can often involve changes in skin oiliness.

## 859 SELECT SELENIUM

The body only needs selenium in tiny amounts but it is crucial for preventing disease, boosting the immune system and helping the skin stay hydrated and undamaged. Selenium protects against toxicity from heavy metals in pollution and works as a healing antioxidant.

## 860 E MAY BE WHAT YOU NEED

Vitamin E is perhaps the body's most important antioxidant, which prevents damage from sun, pollution and modern lifestyles caused by free radicals and oxidation. It has been shown to help skin stay young and healthy looking.

## 861 PINE FOR PERFECT SKIN

Another of nature's very own antioxidants, utilizing the natural protective enzymes and antioxidants of the French pine tree, pine bark extract is an excellent supplement to maintain skin health.

## 862 IMEDEEN FOR AGEING

A natural nutritional supplement containing bio-marine ingredients, vitamin C and zinc, Imedeen nourishes the skin from within to combat the signs of ageing, such as wrinkles, age spots and dry, weak skin.

## 863 WISH UPON A STAR

Starflower oil, extracted from the herb borage, is thought to be even more effective than evening primrose oil because of its incredibly high levels of gamma linoleic acid (GLA), an essential ingredient for skin health.

## 864 THE GENUINE ARTICHOKE

Artichoke is one of the oldest medicinal plants for detoxifying the skin and body. Artichoke leaf extract, containing a chemical called cynarin, stimulates the production of digestive enzymes to help break down food and encourage the release of toxins.

# beauty emergencies

### 865 DIMINISH UNDER-EYE BAGS

For a great solution to firm up under-eye bags and wrinkles, follow the A-list and invest in some haemorrhoid cream, which firms up and tightens skin in delicate areas.

### 866 COPE WITH A HANGOVER

Alcohol is the number one dehydrator and if you're feeling the effects of a hangover, so will your skin. As well as drinking water and steering clear of caffeine, carbonated drinks and juice (diluted juice is fine), help yourself back to humanity with a deep-moisturizing face mask and a rest.

### 867 BANISH GREEN WITH KETCHUP

Blonde hair that's been tinged green from the copper and chlorine in swimming pools can be treated with a good dose of tomato ketchup – apply it from the roots to the tips and leave on for ten minutes, then rinse off for instant colour correction.

## 868 ESCAPE RED-EYE

Red eyes, especially if they're dry, can be a symptom of low vitamin A. Boost your eye health with betacarotene, found in red, orange and yellow fruit and vegetables. Use 'artificial tears' to ease redness. Eyedrops that contain a vasoconstrictor to shrink blood vessels are only a short-term answer and may lead to worsening red eyes.

## 869 BAD HAIR DAYS

Everyone's had them. If you can't get your locks under control or the weather's wreaked havoc with your style, try a ponytail or casual up-do. A little serum or styling cream to slick back the hair can result in a perfectly passable tidy look, even if it's not your best one.

## 870 TEST YOUR IODINE

If you have coarse hair, dry skin and suffer from tiredness, you may be experiencing low iodine levels. Seafood and seaweed are the best sources, or ask your doctor for an iodine test if you're really worried.

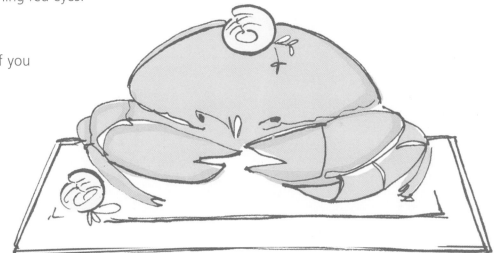

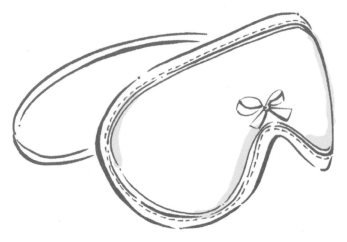

## 873 SMOOTH A BLOTCHY TAN

There is only one real solution for an unevenly applied fake tan – exfoliate, exfoliate, exfoliate. If you don't have the time to invest, try a tan remove; even if it's not the brand of your fake tan, it should neutralize some of the colour.

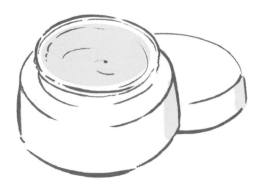

## 871 DE-PUFF UNDER-EYE BAGS

If you wake up in the morning with puffy, swollen eyes, apply a gel-based under-eye product to de-puff the tender skin around your eyes, followed by a cool compress – eye masks, which can be kept in the fridge overnight, are a great choice.

## 872 DON'T BE A RED-RIMMED SPECTACLE

Lack of vitamin C can lead to styes and inflammation and redness of the rims and whites of the eyes. Rich sources are citrus fruits and juices, kiwis, strawberries, broccoli and potatoes.

## 874 POWDER IT OUT

As a quick solution to greasy or oily hair, particularly around the forehead, a dab of translucent powder along the hairline can soak up excess moisture and tide you over until you hit the shower.

## 875 GLOSS OVER EMERGENCIES

Always keep an emergency lip gloss in your handbag. For those sudden meetings or dates, a subtly coloured gloss is the perfect way to dress up your mouth without going over the top.

## 876 COMB AND DRY

If your lashes look more clumpy than naturally dark and luscious, don't wet them in the hope of removing your mascara – the mascara will just clog. Comb through dry lashes with an eyelash comb.

## 877 ROSY CHEEKS

When you don't have enough time to apply make-up, but you don't want to be seen naked-faced, rosy up your cheeks with a quick slick of cream blusher for a naturally beautiful glow.

## 878 FLICK AWAY FLECKS

If your mascara has spread or splattered onto your upper cheeks, dust translucent powder lightly over the cheeks to pick up any mascara flecks.

## 879 TURN ON THE NUDES

To even out self-tan streaks or blotches on the face, use a tinted moisturizer, but avoid any cheek colour or bronzer – instead choose neutral eye and lip colours so that your look is as fresh as possible and you aren't drawing attention to the face.

## 880 ICE THOSE COLD SORES

If you feel the tingling sensation of a cold sore, treat the area with ice immediately, which can help reduce the inflammation around the site and stop the sore from developing. Once the sore has erupted, dab it with salt and lemon.

## 881 BIG SQUEEZE

You've squeezed a spot and it's red and inflamed. Now what? Apply antibacterial ointment and wait for the area to dry. Then apply concealer to the red area and over the base of the spot. Avoid covering up a spot with loose powder before it's dry as the powder can cause the spot to turn crusty – wait until the blemish has stopped weeping first.

### 882 START SMALL

If you suffer eyeshadow creasing, use a small eyeshadow brush with a very small amount of colour and apply in layers to avoid over-doing it. Avoid cream shadows, which have a greater tendency to crease.

### 883 FIX WITH POWDER

To fix creased eyeshadow, apply translucent powder under a powder shadow or over a cream-based one. Wrap your index finger in a tissue and gently remove any residue.

### 884 HIDE TANNING MISTAKES

If you're out and about in the evening, a light-reflecting product will help even out skin tone and disguise any major streaks caused by badly applied self-tan.

### 885 GLOW EVEN WHEN YOU'RE LOW

Apply bronzer lightly across your forehead and under your cheekbones to add a healthy sheen to hungover or over-tired skin, which will help you feel brighter and will stop everyone at work commenting on how tired you look.

### 886 HORROR HAIR COLOUR

If you hate your colour, do not ever try to correct it yourself with an at-home dye or go to an alternative hairdresser. Immediately return to the original stylist, tell them you are unhappy and ask if they can remedy the situation. They prefer happy clients, so will usually comply, free of charge, and you won't be throwing good money after bad.

### 887 GET SALTY

Reduce your chances of infection in cuts and broke skin using salt to cleanse and detoxify small wounds. Or sprinkle a pinch of turmeric onto cuts to boost the skin's natural healing process. To stop bleeding from a shaving nick, use a styptic pencil but if you don't have one, try a tiny dab of anti-perspirant, alcohol or peroxide.

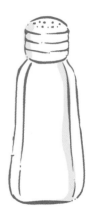

## 889 PENCIL IT IN

To correct over-plucked eyebrows, choose an eyebrow pencil as close to your brow colour as possible and lightly pencil in, following your natural line. Use short pencil strokes, then brush out your brow to soften the line.

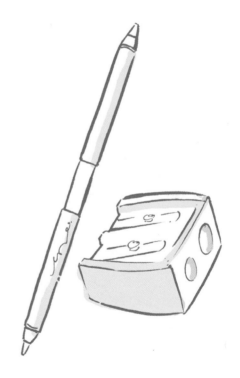

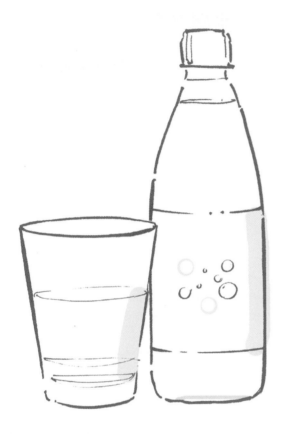

## 888 WATER IT WELL

If your skin looks pale and your eyes dull, this could be the first signs of dehydration, and simply topping up your water levels could give your looks a boost.

# 890 TRY THE TOOTHPASTE TRICK

If you suddenly find you have a spot the night before a big party or interview, apply toothpaste to it overnight, which will help dry out the skin and reduce redness around the area.

# 891 SMALL IS BEAUTIFUL

Cover a problem spot with a small, pointy brush dipped in concealer and paint it out – a tiny brush allows you to target the blemish without making the cover-up attempt obvious. Choose a brush with a lid so you can retouch the spot easily.

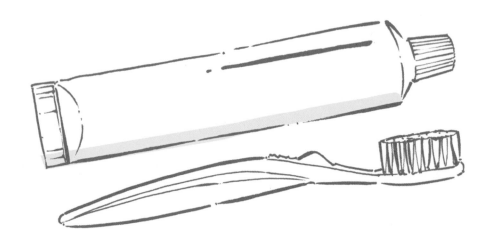

**892** **HAVE A CUPPA FOR PUFFY EYES**

For soothing and reducing puffiness in tired, swollen eyes, soak a couple of tea bags in warm water. Squeeze them until just damp and rest for ten minutes with the tea bags on closed eyes. Tea's natural antioxidant properties will get to work on your problem.

**893** **PRIME SKIN WITH POST-LUNCH POWDER**

After lunch the skin on your face can often become shiny and greasy. Dust on an oil-free powder to cut out the shine, but don't go overboard; just stick to a thin layer and reapply the powder later if necessary.

**894** **WIPE UP AFTER WORKOUTS**

Even if you don't feel like you've sweated much during exercise, chances are your skin has evaporated more moisture. For a quick fix post-exercise, when you don't have time for a full shower, use cleansing wipes to remove sweat and oil. Clean skin will reduce the chance of blemishes and keep the pores clear.

## 895 FIX UP A SHAKY FOUNDATION

Like energy levels, foundation can flag by four o' clock in the afternoon, but a five-minute bathroom touch-up will do the trick. First, blot your face to get rid of excess oil and then blend in foundation that has creased using a clean make-up sponge. Dust translucent powder all over and swipe on a subtle blush and lipstick.

## 896 TAKE THE SPONGE

If there's one thing you should carry with you in case of beauty emergencies, it's a packet of clean cosmetic sponges, which can be used to smooth out or reapply foundation, blend creased eyeshadow and blend streaky areas.

## 897 BRONZE AWAY BLEARY EYES

If your skin and eyes are suffering from a lack of sleep, a bronze- or gold-coloured eyeliner or shadow placed near the lash line is the quickest way to make you look wide awake and perky. Bronze is the best universal eye brightener, working with most colours of eyes.

## 898 LIP UP YOUR CHEEKS

When you're caught looking pale or tired with nothing on you but a lipstick, use a few dabs on your cheeks, blended in with fingers, to give yourself a healthy glow.

# big day... & night

## 899 FIRST THINGS FIRST

For big nights out you want your eye make-up to last until the wee hours. To provide a good base, first apply foundation on your eyelids only, and then apply your eyeshadow. When done, lightly mist water over your eyes to set. Then apply the rest of your foundation and make-up as usual.

## 900 GO WARM ON BRIDAL LIPS

Brides should choose a lip colour in a warm, fairly bright shade. Roses, pinks and reds look great in photos and keep teeth and wedding whites looking clean and fresh.

## 901 BE LAVISH WITH LASHES

Create lush lashes by using an eyelash curler and applying two thin coats of lengthening mascara. Don't overwhelm your lashes with too many coats, especially if your big moment is in the daytime, because your lashes can look clumpy and there's more chance of fall-out. Waterproof mascara is longlasting and won't run if you shed a few tears of joy.

## 902 GET A PROFESSIONAL LOOK

Head to your nearest make-up counter or boutique for a special consultation. Not only will they be able to show you great colours, but they'll also give you tips on techniques and insider tricks as well. Sometimes high-profile make-up artists make store visits so keep an eye out for any advertisement giving dates and times for these free events.

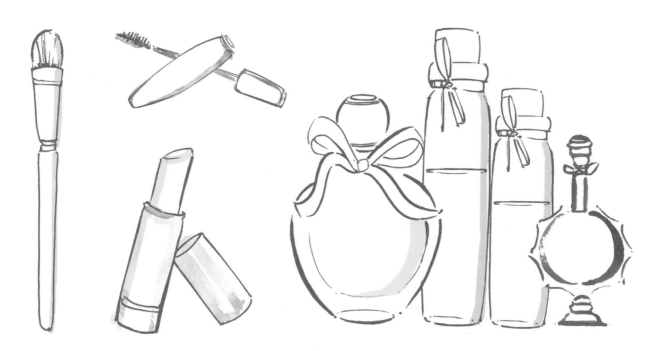

## 903 GO WARM ON CHEEKS

For wedding days, when you naturally want to emphasize your youth and beauty, choose a warm, flattering cheek colour in a pinky peach or rose, which will look like a natural extension of your skin tone. Focus on the rounded parts of the cheek and blend the blush back and up toward your hairline.

## 904 TEST WHAT LOOKS BEST

Always try at least one test-run of what you'd like to look like on your big day – with full dress, hair and make-up. Do it a few weeks before the big event and time yourself so that you know to leave enough time on the day itself. For make-up, think about what time of day you want to make your best impression, and don't be afraid to change your look if the occasion runs from day into evening, adding some darker colours or sparkle if you are going to be dancing later on.

# 905 DON'T FOLLOW FASHION

Don't get too trendy with your eye make-up on your wedding day. You may think that sparkly eyeliner is a good idea today, but chances are you'll look back at the pictures years from now and regret it. Keep it natural and fresh and be wary of using a make-up artist who doesn't know you well – they could make your look too strong or too pale for you, and you'll spend needless time retouching your face.

# 906 AVOID THE BURN

Don't get too much sun before a big event. Sunburns, peeling skin and tan lines can sabotage your special day because they're difficult to cover up completely.

# 907 UP-DO HAIR-DO

For a wedding day, black-tie event or other formal occasion, try a sleek sophisticated chignon. Visit your hairdresser for a trial run first to see how it will look and whether it will suit your dress. Your stylist will be able to advise on using hairpieces and aids to achieve the look you want.

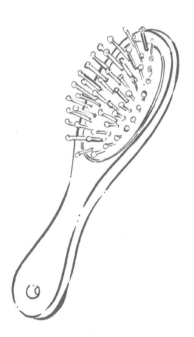

### 908 KEEP YOUR FACE ON

Give your foundation staying power by using a gel foundation primer before you apply your make-up. Add a light dusting of loose powder to prevent any unwanted shine.

# holiday beauty

### 909 STAY ABOVE THE CUT

Before you go on a beach holiday, take a trip to the hairdresser for a pre-holiday trim. Damaged ends will only get worse when exposed to the drying effects of sun, salt and chlorine, so make sure you set off with your hair in tiptop form.

### 910 CARRY ON CAMPING

Space is at a premium in a tent so you won't want to take your usual bottles of cleanser and toner. Extra-mild baby wipes are a brilliant substitute, even for removing stubborn mascara, and can be helpful for many other cleaning tasks.

### 911 STROLL IN THE SEA

Give your bum and thighs a workout by strolling in water that's at least knee deep. It will keep you cool in the sun and, because you're working against resistance, help tone up your legs and bottom.

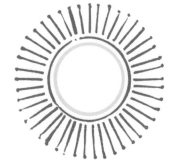

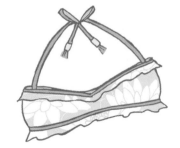

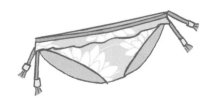

## 912 BE A GLOSS ADJUSTER

Before you go away, protect your hair using a semi-permanent gloss colour treatment, which will not only make you feel great but also adds a layer of protection to your hair, preventing it from moisture loss. To really bolster hair health, treat yourself to a deep-conditioning treatment, either using a rich cream mask or a treatment oil to boost moisture and gleam.

## 913 PLAIT IT UP

If you have long hair, consider putting it into a plait when you're on the beach or by the pool – this will reduce the amount of hair (especially ends) which are in contact with the sun's damaging rays and help your hair stay looking healthy.

## 914 CURL AND DYE

Have your lashes curled and dyed before you jet off to the beach and you won't have to worry about waterproof mascara or panda eyes. Tints have the added bonus of swelling your lashes, making them appear thicker.

## 915 SKI AWAY TO BEAUTY

Cold mountain air and high altitudes can wreak havoc with moisture levels, so be sure to drink as much water as you can. Avoid astringents or clay face masks, which are drying. Instead of foundation, cover blemishes and red areas with concealer and use a copious amount of sunblock, paying particular attention to the hairline and ears.

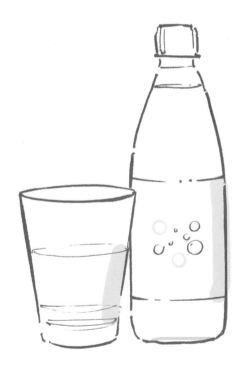

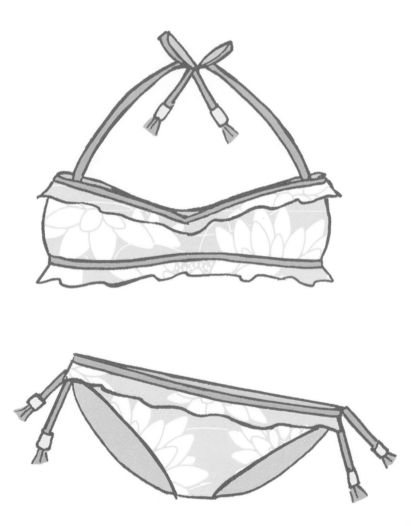

### 916 BE SHORE-FOOTED

Walking on sand is one of the best ways to naturally exfoliate your feet and reduce foot tension, as the hard grains give you a massage and pedicure at the same time!

### 917 PRICKLY PAIR

If you find yourself suffering from prickly heat – small red bumps on the skin that itch severely – wear natural fibres like cotton and linen, and don't be tempted to scratch, which will make it worse. Products containing salicylic acid can help.

### 918 VISIT AN EXPERT

If your hair has suffered while you were away, pay a trip to your hairdresser as soon as you get back for a quick trim to remove damaged ends. That way, the damage and splits won't spread up the hair shafts.

### 919 PREVENT BITES WITH COAL TAR

Using coal tar soap to wash yourself in the bath or shower can help keep biting insects at bay, so you don't arrive home from your holiday covered in bites and itchy marks.

# picture perfect

### 920 SIGH AWAY CHINS, LOOK BLINKS AWAY

To avoid double chins in photographs, take a deep breath just before the shutter goes down and sigh out as you smile or pose, which will tighten the area under the chin and avoid it sagging. If you tend to blink in photos, look down or to the side, and just before the photographer is ready to take the shot, move your eyes back to the camera.

### 921 FIND AN INTERESTING ANGLE

Look at photos of yourself that you like and try to replicate your position in the future. Many people look better with their head slightly angled to the side than straight on.

### 922 USE CONTRAST

Photography, especially if there's a flash involved, can wash out pale colours. To prepare for important photographs, consider putting on a little more make-up than normal to ensure you look your best.

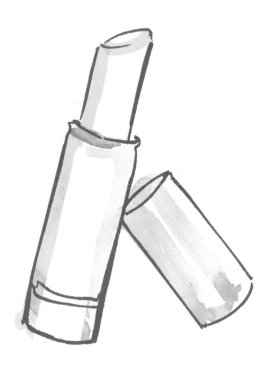

### 923 AVOID FROSTING

For photos, never make the mistake of wearing a lipstick that is too neutral or frosted. These colours can leave you looking pale or tired and will wash out your face.

### 924 SIMMER ON THE SHIMMER

Don't get carried away with shimmer highlighters. In photos, these can give you an unflattering and highly reflective shine, which may look very overdone. Aim for subtlety.

### 925 SIDE ON

For a slimming standing pose, copy the celebrities and hold your body at a three-quarter pose with one foot in front of the other and with your arms held away from your body – this will minimize the amount of space your body takes up and make your extremities look leaner. Stand tall with the shoulders back. At the moment before the picture is taken, tuck your bottom in slightly – this thrusts the hips out a little and makes your torso look longer.

## 926 DON'T DRESS TO IMPRESS

Don't use a heavy pressed powder to set your foundation if you want to look your best in photographs. Too much powder can leave your skin looking chalky and dull.

## 927 GO YELLOW IN A FLASH

Foundations with slightly yellow undertones work best with flash photography, so be careful with rose tones which can look harsh and make you appear red in the face.

## 928 BE EDGY

For sitting photographs, move to the edge of your chair so your thighs drop down rather than spread out and look larger than they actually are.

## 929 GET SIDEWAYS

In groups, don't be the one caught in the middle with both your arms around the others, which can make you look wider as you are facing the camera straight on. Instead, use one arm around another person and keep the other arm low.

## 930 THINGS ARE LOOKING UP

If someone is taking a shot of your face and you want your cheeks to look slimmer, ask them to take it from above you. Looking up at the camera will widen your eyes and narrow your cheeks. A quick trick to avoid the appearance of a double chin is to touch your tongue to the roof of your mouth.

## 931 DON'T BE BROWBEATEN

Remember that photos increase contrast, so don't use dark shadows or pencils to define your brows, as this may leave you looking stern rather than stunning. Likewise too much kohl eyeliner and smoky eyeshadows can create dark pools in the eye area, making your eyes appear much more deeply set.

## 932 THE LOWDOWN ON LOOKING GOOD

Unless you're super tall, never let anyone take a full-length photo of you from eye level, as this will shorten your legs. Ask them to squat on the ground and aim up for a more flattering leg-lengthening angle.

# seasonal beauty

## 933 BEWARE OF SPOTS

Spots are more common in spring than winter, as the skin begins to produce the oils it has been lacking over the dry winter months. Cleanse day and night and switch your moisturizer to a light formula.

## 934 STEAM AHEAD

Once a week during the spring months treat your facial skin to at-home herbal steam therapy using Ayurvedic powders or homemade versions by steeping garden herbs in boiling water. This will help to rejuvenate the skin's natural detox process.

## 935 PREPARE TO BARE

It's not just the skin on your face which needs attention in spring. Most likely, your body has been covered up during the winter months, so make sure you welcome it back to exposure with all-over exfoliation and moisturization.

## 936 LESS IS MORE IN SUMMERTIME

If you change one thing with the seasons, make it your base. Winter foundation will look dull and heavy in the summer, when the light is brighter and your skin is a different colour. Switch to a lighter formula, a tinted moisturizer or just use concealer and a sunscreen.

## 937 HIT THE WATER BOTTLE

Drink lots of water throughout the day during summer months, not only to replenish moisture lost to the heat and sweat, but also to help flush toxins out of the body and keep skin looking clear and lustrous. Herb or spice teas, made with skin-enhancing ingredients, offer added therapeutic benefits.

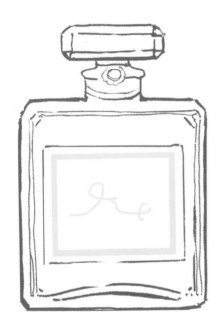

## 938 LIGHTEN YOUR SCENTS

Choose a light formula of fragrance for the summer months – an eau de toilette or a body spritz in the floral or ozonic family is more refreshing and suitable than the autumnal woody and spicy chypre and fougère fragrances.

## 939 TAKE A WALK ON THE MILD SIDE

If you want to enjoy the sun, go easy on spicy and very sour foods, like chilli, lime and vinegar, which may increase skin's reactivity to sunlight and cause irritation. Stick to milder foods with high water content instead.

## 940 MILK IT

Milk has cooling properties, which supply nutrients to the skin and keep it from drying out by assisting in forming a protective layer against water loss. Drink a glass of milk every day in hot weather, or choose cleansers and moisturizers with milk added.

## 941 BEAT THE OIL

The sun can increase sebum production, causing your skin to look oily on occasion. When the oil combines with dirt and sweat, pores get clogged. In summer, you must be meticulous about your cleansing routine, morning and night, especially if you're using sun-blocking creams. If you really suffer from oily skin, avoid night-time moisturizers to give your skin a break.

## 942 MASK THE PROBLEM

Once a week during summer, use a face mask derived from fruit to help rebalance and rejuvenate summer skin, removing excess oils without drying. Avocado, cucumber and papaya are all great fruit mask choices.

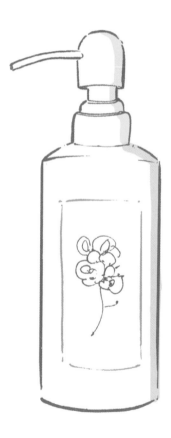

## 943 DEVOTE TIME TO YOUR DECOLLETAGE

The skin on your chest and neck is almost as delicate as that on your face, but it's easily forgotten in the autumn, when you're likely to start covering up more. Apply a moisturizer at night on your neck, ears and collarbone area, as well as your face to keep it toned.

## 944 BE CLUED UP ABOUT CLEANSERS

Autumn brings with it colder weather, which means the oils the skin has been producing liberally throughout the warmth of the summer begin to fade. Make sure autumn cleansers are free from detergents which could strip the skin of moisture.

## 945 A COMPACT SOLUTION

Even dry skins can shine in the summer. Take a powder compact with you at all times to correct the extra shine and you may even be able to forgo foundation or tinted moisturizer entirely. Fight bacteria by using a make-up brush for dabbing on the powder, rather than the pad applicator that comes with the compact.

## 946 GO YELLOW

Be aware that summer light has more yellow tones to it than winter's grey. Choose your tones carefully and make sure you check your make-up in daylight before you venture out. Look out for sallow areas around eyes and neck.

## 947 REMEMBER THE SUN

Even though the sun may no longer be generating high summer heat, don't take that as a sign to throw away your sun block. Dermatologists now recommend an SPF of 15–30 for all skin types in summer, and 15–20 during autumn to prevent sun damage.

## 948 BE A PLUM FAIRY

Instead of immediately opting for dark colours in the autumn, step slowly into winter with deep berry colours, plums and slate greys, which blend with summer skin and brighten dark autumn nights. Simply choosing a different shade of lipstick can be enough to direct your look toward the new season.

## 949 DON'T BE HOT TO TROT

The thought of a long, hot bath on a cold, winter day can be appealing, but over-exposure to hot water can dry skin out even more. Keep baths or showers short, limit them to one per day and use warm, not hot, water.

## 950 GO HOT AND COLD

Start the winter's day with a warm shower but, before you get out, switch to cold water for about 15 seconds, then turn the water from cold to hot and back a few times to stimulate sluggish circulation and to invigorate the skin.

## 951 GET RICH QUICK

Use a rich daily moisturizer to keep skin plumped up and well oiled during winter months when it can often become dry and dull. This will help it retain a healthy glow. If possible, avoid AHAs, retinol products and strong exfoliators that strip away your skin in winter and look for enriching ingredients such as vitamin E, amino acids, hyaluronic acid that will quench dry skin.

## 952 NO TIME TO CHAP

Chapped lips are often the most noticeable problem when it comes to dryness in the winter. Use a highly moisturizing lip balm, which provides a protective barrier, with vitamin E for good elasticity.

## 953 SCRUB UP WELL

Exfoliate once a week to remove dead skin cells and allow the skin to absorb extra moisture, which is lost from the skin's lower layers during winter because of harsher, cooler temperatures. It will help your skin stay pink and glowing rather than grey and dull.

## 954 WAKE UP WITH WATER AND LEMON

This Chinese herbal remedy is a sure-fire method of energizing your body. It will detox your entire system, including the liver and gall bladder, which means your body will be able to clean the blood faster to rid itself of the toxins responsible for poor skin. Simply add a few slices of fresh lemon or the juice of half a lemon to a cup of hot water and drink it.

## 955 COME ON STRONG

Dull colours in winter mean thickening up make-up looks great. Go for black rather than the beiges and browns of summer, and risk metallic shades and darker lips, which will smoulder in winter's flatter light.

## 956 GO MILD

Throw away soap, which can irritate drier skin, and switch to a milder, gentler cleanser for face and body. Soap can irritate and exacerbate dry skin conditions. Instead of rubbing yourself dry, pat to remove excess moisture.

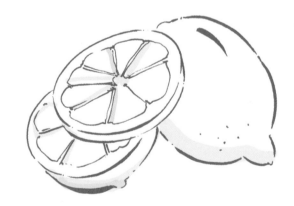

## 957 TAKE MATTERS IN HAND

Pay extra attention to hands and feet in winter, when skin can crack and peel. Always apply hand cream after you wash your hands and limit exposure to water by wearing rubber gloves for washing up and cleaning.

## 958 AIM FOR SPF8

Unless you're skiing, you don't need a high SPF during the winter, when the sunlight is weaker. Change down from an SPF 15 to an 8 to give your skin a chance to absorb vitamin D and avoid developing sensitivity to the chemicals in sunscreens.

## 959 PLAY INDOOR BOWLS

To combat the drying effects of central heating, place houseplants in your home and office (and water or mist them frequently). For an instant humidifier in the bedroom, place a bowl of water near a radiator or heat source to keep moisture levels high in the room and aid respiration overnight.

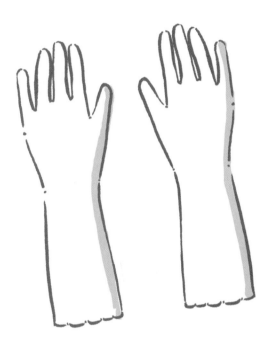

# travel

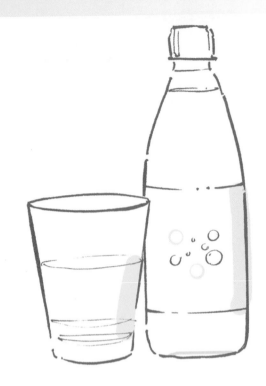

## 960 BE A WATER BABY

For every hour onboard a flight, you can lose 100 ml (3½ fl oz) of water from your skin. Keep hydrated by drinking at least 250 ml (8½ fl oz) of water every hour and moisturize your face and body well before flying.

## 961 SAFE LANDINGS

Post-flight skin is usually tired and dehydrated, so using lots of make-up to make yourself look better won't help. Instead, apply moisturizer and smudge cheeks with colour-enhancing cream blush or gel bronzer. Use an oil or moisturizer containing vitamin E, which will help beat sagginess and give skin a plumper feel.

## 962 MILK IT UP

Taking a supplement of milk thistle if you're travelling abroad will help aid digestion, protect against stomach bugs, boost your immune system and help your liver deal with holiday excess.

## 963 WAKE YOURSELF UP

Humidity is usually less than 20 per cent in airplanes. To freshen dehydrated skin and eyes on longhaul flights, splash your face with cold water and apply plenty of light, non-clogging moisturizer and an eye cream. This will tone the skin and enliven puffy eyes. Spritzing the face with a rosewater atomizer during the flight will also help keep skin supple and soft.

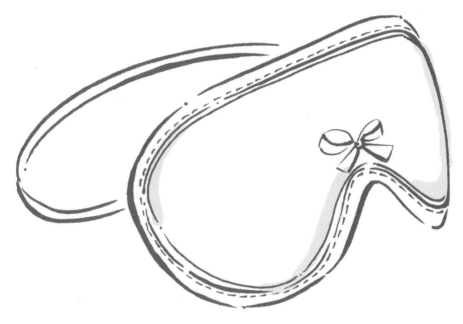

## 964 SLEEP IN THE CLOUDS

The best thing you can do on a plane is to
sleep as much as you can. Get comfortable
by using a neck pillow, as this area of the
body is the one most prone to stiffness after
a flight. Invest in an eye mask and ear plugs
to block out excess light and noise,
whatever the distractions.

### 965 USE A FACE TREATMENT

Instead of accepting that flying will make your skin look bad, fight off dullness by using a face treatment while you're on board, particularly on your cheeks, which are often the first areas to show telltale signs of dehydration like fine lines.

### 966 TRAVEL WITH A TINT

Tinted moisturizer is an excellent product for travelling. Not only is it easy to transport and apply, but it can work equally well as a moisturizer, foundation and SPF all in one. It's also less drying than many foundations, which is a must for dehydrated skin.

### 967 MULTITASK YOUR MAKE-UP

Triple crayons and multi-use products like lip and cheek stains are great for travelling because you can apply them on the go with fingers for a quick boost and they take up precious little space in your handbag. Vaseline also makes a great moisturizer, lip balm, highlighter and first-aid salve.

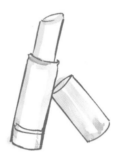
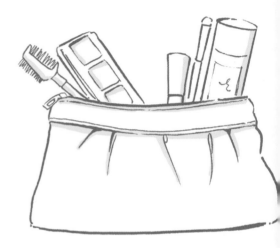

### 968 GLOSS IT UP

If you're travelling to warmer climes, lipstick sometimes seems too chalky or heavy. Instead, take a lipliner and lip gloss in your handbag. Line lightly or colour in the whole lip for an instant natural boost that will stay on your lips for hours.

## 969 PACK IN THE BOX

Instead of carrying a handful of lipsticks with you on holiday, invest in a pill case and fill the sections with different lip shades. Not only have you created your own lip palette, you'll also be able to leave the rest at home, preventing heat damage.

## 970 USE UP YOUR FREEBIES

Take any extra free trial-size products from magazines or beauty counters with you. Don't be afraid to ask for samples at beauty counters – in addition to providing good miniature-sizes for travelling and weekends away, it will enable you to try out a product first before investing in a costly purchase for the full-size item.

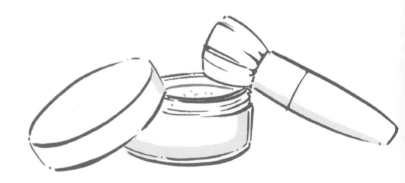

## 971 FLEX THE FEET

For a quick exercise during a train, car or plane journey where you will be stationary for some time, stand on one foot and bend the other behind you, grasping the ankle in your hand. Now flex and unflex your foot – this will keep the blood flowing and help prevent thrombosis and pins and needles.

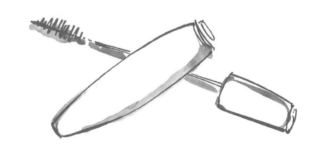

## 972 DON'T TOIL WITH YOUR TOILETRIES

Decant your everyday supplies into plastic bottles to take with you – this will avoid any glass breakages and ensure that your toiletry kit is user-friendly and lightweight.

## 973 CLEANSE WITH CLOTHS

Always pack cleansing cloths for a long flight, which will help you keep skin clean and clog-free throughout your journey. Follow with moisturizer to prevent the skin from drying out, and you'll arrive looking as bright-faced as ever.

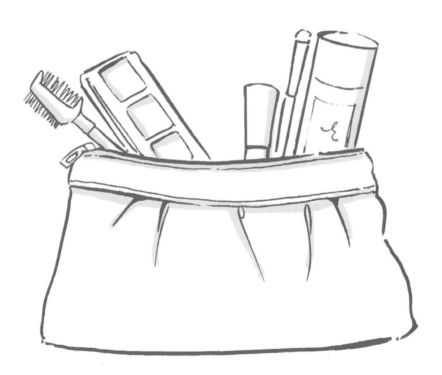

## 974 VANITY CASE

Keep everything at home that you can, taking only the essentials with you. Look for multiple-use products, such as cleansers that double as moisturizers, body lotions that are also formulated for hair conditioning and shea butter balm that conditions nails, hands and lips. A palette of lip, eye and cheek colours will take up much less space than individual products.

## 975 BE BOLD WITH BRONZER

Travelling often makes skin look tired and dull. Bronzer is a great all-round product for warming up pale skin and gives you a glow. It can also be used as a blush or eyeshadow for a more grown-up look.

## 976 BRIGHTEN UP

To instantly enliven a tired face, blend a bit of illuminizer or radiance booster over the centre of the chin, the bridge of the nose and the middle of the forehead, which will help give the appearance of a natural, vital glow. If your neck or shoulders are bare, add a little there, too.

# yummy mummies

## 977 BANISH BRUISES WITH MARIGOLD

Pregnant skin is more prone to bruising. Make a bruise-busting infusion with a handful of marigold (*calendula officianalis*) flowers and 300 ml (½ pint) of boiled water. Steep for five minutes, allow to cool, then wipe the bruised area. Arnica cream is a good homeopathic alternative.

## 978 CHOOSE CREAM CAREFULLY

The best creams to prevent stretch marks from occurring are those that contain collagen and elastin, which help regenerate the skin's lower layers and reduce the chances of it being stretched and scarred.

## 979 E-RASE STRETCH MARKS

Use vitamin E cream on stretch marks, massaging it into delicate or affected areas once or twice a day to make them less visible and to prevent others appearing in the first place.

### 980 BE PATIENT WITH PIGMENT CHANGES

Some women suffer marked pigment changes on their face in pregnancy – called chloasma – because of hormonal changes. If you suffer from this, avoid the sun (which makes it worse) and use make-up to even out your skin tone. Your complexion should revert to normal a few months after the baby is born.

### 981 SWIM WELL AS YOU SWELL

Swimming is one of the best exercises for pregnancy because all the body is supported, but chlorine and chemicals can strip skin of moisture and leave it feeling dull and dry. Make sure you use rich body lotions to counteract the drying effects.

### 982 MASSAGE YOUR BUMP

Skin is under a great deal of pressure during pregnancy, with a lot of stretching to do, especially in the abdominal area. Massaging your bump with oil, cream or gel will keep skin supple and elastic, and boost circulation. This will also provide relief if you suffer from an itchy belly.

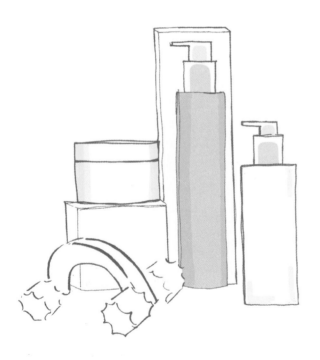

## 983 CHANGE PRODUCTS

When you're pregnant, hormones cause changes and sensitivity in your natural skin and hair, so reconsider the suitability of your normal products, which may not be the best to use at this time.

## 984 FEED HUNGRY SKIN

The turnover of skin cells is accelerated during pregnancy as the metabolic rate increases, so make sure you nourish and moisturize more than normal to keep skin looking healthy. Concentrate on areas that expand, like the breasts and abdomen. Choose moisturizers that are as pure as possible, such as cocoa butter, as everything you put on your skin has a chance of being absorbed into the bloodstream.

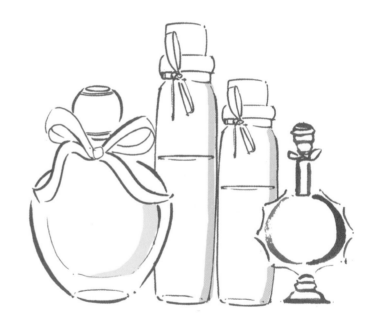

## 985 LOVE YOUR CURVES

Instead of worrying about your growing curves, make the most of them with softer hair and make-up for a more feminine look. It's only nine months, after all, and the sooner you accept your new curves, the more you'll enjoy them!

### 986 FAKE TAN MAKES MARKS FAINT

Fake tan will help conceal stretch marks by colouring the skin and minimizing their visibility. This trick is especially good for silvery pink marks. Real tanning, however, makes stretchmarks more obvious, so stay out of the sun.

### 987 FEED YOUR FEET

Feet can get tired and swollen in pregnancy as the body copes with high levels of blood and fluid circulating in the body. A refreshing foot gel with menthol will really pep you up at the end of a long day, especially if you rest with your feet up.

### 988 STAND TALL

With all the changes in weight and gravity that your body goes through as part of a normal pregnancy, your back may tend to slouch. Try to keep your hips in line with your shoulders rather than pushing them forward as you stand or walk. Good posture will not only help you look taller and less dumpy but will evenly distribute the strain of the added baby weight.

### 989 RETREAT FROM RETIN-A

Increased androgen levels make women more prone to blemishes during the first three months of pregnancy, but you should avoid using acne medications which may cause harm to the developing foetus. These include vitamin A-derivative lotions such as Accutane and Retin-A.

### 990 DON'T REACH OILING POINT

If your skin suffers from oiliness during pregnancy, particularly on your face, make sure your cleansers, moisturizers and suncreams are labelled as non-comedogenic (not pore-blocking) and non-acnegenic (not spot-causing).

### 991 EXTEND YOUR EXFOLIATION

Skin regenerates itself more quickly during pregnancy, which means dead skin cells are more likely to build up on the surface, causing dullness and spots. Thoroughly cleanse your face morning and night and use a gentle exfoliator on the face and body two or three times a week to keep skin soft, clear and uncongested.

## 992 EXTREMITIES NEED EXTRA CARE

Skin on the hands, feet, lower legs and arms is often neglected by the circulation system during pregnancy, as the body concentrates on the growing baby. Gentle exercises and massage can help encourage blood flow to the area to counteract dryness and tingling sensations.

## 993 FACE UP TO THE NEW YOU

Many women's face shapes change during pregnancy, becoming fuller and more rounded. Rather than lamenting it, ask your hairdresser to suggest subtle changes to your hair to flatter your new look – straight, shoulder-length hair can help slim cheeks, for example.

## 994 CUT DOWN ON CHEMICALS

Instead of using chemical products or straighteners to create a smooth look, which might affect the baby, dry your hair straight using a straightening balm, a natural bristle brush and a nozzled hairdryer. Alternatively, try a light-hold gel to keep natural curls tamed.

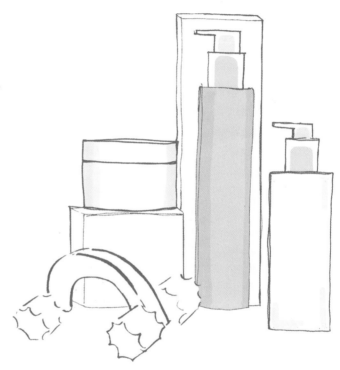

## 995 BABY KNOWS BEST

Mild baby products are suitable for sensitive skin that is going through hormonal upheavals, so raid your child's supply of baby oil, shampoo and talcum powder. Choose unscented varieties.

# 996 IT MAKES SCENTS

Make the most of your heightened sense of smell and give yourself a lift by spritzing on a clean, fresh scent. Choose a light floral or ozonic fragrance that won't overpower you or make you feel nauseous.

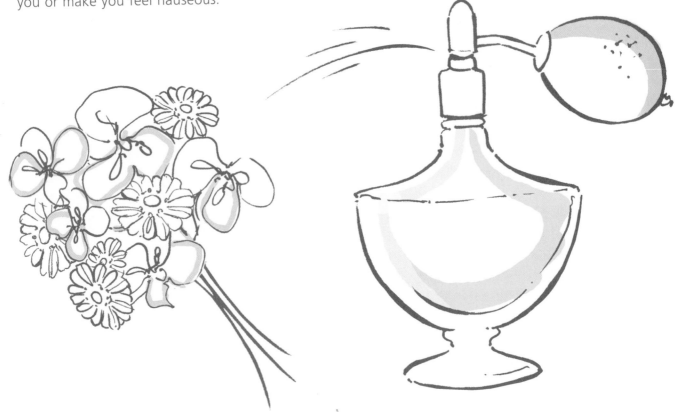

## 987 COUNT TO THREE

Most doctors and hair stylists recommend not submitting your hair to any chemical processes during the first three months of pregnancy because of extra sensitivity to chemical fumes. This includes colouring, perming or chemical straightening. Even after this, always seek professional advice, as there is ongoing debate as to whether the processes are safe for the baby. To make safe hair colour changes, try a hair wand, gel or mascara, which give a temporary non-toxic colour highlight that only lasts as long as your next wash.

## 988 GO VEGGIE

Any hair colouring process should avoid touching the skin and scalp to prevent the absorption of chemicals into the bloodstream during pregnancy. To be safe, opt for highlights and streaks which do not touch the scalp, instead of all-over colour. Rather than your usual bleach or ammonia highlights while pregnant, ask for vegetable dyes or use henna, which do not contain chemicals.

## 999 IT'S HARD NOT TO DRY

Breastfeeding can make hair very dry, as the body directs most of its nutrients towards the baby. It should return to normal once you stop, but an extra-moisturizing shampoo and deep conditioner will help until then.

## 1000 BEWARE OF THE BARE

One of the biggest beauty mistakes pregnant women make is abandoning cosmetics entirely. Instead, lightly make-up eyes and lips to help you feel like a natural beauty. Because of the increased bloodflow in the body, cheeks often become red and blotchy. Cover them up with a natural-looking foundation or concealer and keep them well moisturized to prevent dry and flaky patches.

## 1001 HEAD FOR A SCARF

Long hair can seem extra hot and bothersome when you're pregnant or in care of a small babe. Keeping locks held back with a fashionable hairband or scarf will allow you to go about your daily jobs in comfort without compromising your sex appeal.

AUTHOR ACKNOWLEDEMENTS
With thanks to:
Paul McEwan, Pauline Floyd,
Jo Philpot and Julia Rogers